Ethics in paed

Ethics in paediatric nursing

Edited by

Gosia M. Brykczyńska

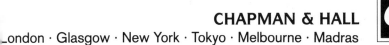

CHAPMAN & HALL

London · Glasgow · New York · Tokyo · Melbourne · Madras

**Published by Chapman & Hall, 2-6 Boundary Row,
London SE1 8HN, UK**

Chapman & Hall, 2-6 Boundary Row, London SE1 8HN, UK

Blackie Academic & Professional, Wester Cleddens Road, Bishopbriggs,
Glasgow G64 2NZ, UK

Chapman & Hall Inc., One Penn Plaza, 41st Floor, New York
NY 10119, USA

Chapman & Hall Japan, Thomson Publishing Japan, Hirakawacho
Nemoto Building, 6F, 1-7-11 Hirakawa-cho, Chiyoda-ku, Tokyo 102,
Japan

Chapman & Hall Australia, Thomas Nelson Australia, 102 Dodds Street,
South Melbourne, Victoria 3205, Australia

Chapman & Hall India, R. Seshadri, 32 Second Main Road, CIT East,
Madras 600 035, India

First edition 1989
Reprinted 1992, 1994

© 1989 Chapman & Hall

Typeset in 10/12pt Sabon by Mayhew Typesetting, Bristol
Printed in Great Britain by St Edmundsbury Press Ltd, Bury St Edmunds,
Suffolk

ISBN 0 412 32960 3

A catalogue record for this book is available from the British Library
Library of Congress Cataloging-in-Publication Data available

Contents

Contents

Appendices:

Contributors

BELINDA ATKINSON RGN,RSCN,DIP.N(LOND)
Services Clinical Manager, Intensive Care Services, Southampton General Hospital, Southampton

GOSIA M. BRYKCZYŃSKA RGN,RSCN,Onc. Cert,RNT,BA,BSc,Cert Ed
Formerly Nurse Teacher, Charles West School of Nursing, Great Ormond Street, London; currently Lecturer/Tutor, Institute of Advanced Nursing Education, St Bartholomew's Hospital, London

PHILIP DARBYSHIRE MN,RNMH,RSCN,DN,RNT
Scottish Home and Health Dept, Nursing Research Training Fellow, Nursing Research Unit, Dept of Nursing Studies, University of Edinburgh, Edinburgh

WALLACE B. HAMILTON RMN,RCNT,Cert Teaching Nurs. Subjects, Cert Child and Adolescent Psychiatric Nursing
Western College of Nursing and Midwifery, Glasgow

MARK WHITING RSCN,DN,SRN,HV,B Nursing,MSc
Community Paediatric Nurse Charge, Community Paediatric Office, Central Middlesex Hospital, London

DOROTHY A. WHYTE RSCN
Lecturer in Nursing Studies, Dept of Nursing Studies, University of Edinburgh, Edinburgh

Acknowledgements

Acknowledgements are given to the following organizations for permission to include their material in the appendices of this book:

- National Association for the Welfare of Children in Hospital, Argyle House, 29–31 Euston Road, London NW1 2SD: *NAWCH Charter for Children in Hospital*.

- UNICEF – United Nations Children's Fund UK Committee, 55 Lincoln's Inn Fields, London WC2A 3NB: *The Declaration of the Rights of the Child*, November 1959.

- ICN – International Council of Nurses, 3, Place Jean-Marteau, CH–1201 Geneva, Switzerland: *ICN Nurses Guidelines for Conduction of Ethical Research* (1977); *ICN Code for Nurses Ethical Concepts Applied to Nursing* (1973).

- UKCC – United Kingdom Central Council for Nursing, Midwifery and Health Visiting, 23 Portland Place, London W1N 3AF: *Code of Professional Conduct*, 2nd edn, November 1984.

- RCN – Society of Paediatric Nursing, 20 Cavendish Square, London W1M 0AB: *Statement of Values in Paediatric Nursing*, August 1987.

Preface

The idea to write a book on ethical issues pertaining to paediatric nursing has been aired for quite some time. The single most significant factor in holding up the creation of such a book was the lack of expertise in one person of all the areas of paediatric nursing. The problem was resolved by producing an edited book, covering various specialities of paediatric nursing. Undoubtedly, one could have included more detailed coverage of particular speciality areas, e.g. chapters on ethical issues surrounding adolescent care, child abuse, teenage mothers, behaviour modification programmes and so on. The approach we took, however, stressed the overall unity of paediatric nursing – where the specialities are wide enough to take in all paediatric nursing activities from neonatal care to adolescent health screening.

I am certainly very aware that the book would not have been written and produced without the support, enthusiasm and co-operation of the chapter-writers. I would also especially like to thank Christine Birdsall, Nursing Editor at Chapman and Hall, and my colleagues at the Charles West School of Nursing – Joanna Parkes and Imelda Charles–Edwards, for their continuing support, and my family and friends, all of whom bore with me during the last two years.

Lastly, I would like to thank Barbara Weller from the Department of Child Health DHSS, for generously agreeing to comment critically on the manuscript and all the students, nurses and children I have met over the years, without whose insights and wisdom I would never have been inspired to pursue the publication of such a book. To all and everyone, thank you for your help and support – or as we say in Polish: bóg zaptać.

Foreword

Ethical issues relating to paediatric nursing were, until the 1980s, frequently presumed to be the domain of medical colleagues or a handful of nursing academics. Discussions focused on life and death ethical issues and few nurses consciously considered the ethical implications of their individual practice.

The recent upsurge in interest, which indicates the professional maturation of nurses, has been influenced by many factors. In the late 1970s, the nursing profession was concerned at what it perceived to be the fallen standards of nursing care; this concern led to the establishment of a Royal College of Nursing (RCN) Committee. The Committee's work led to two publications; Standards of Nursing Care (1980) and Towards Standards (1981) highlighting the paucity of toils with which to measure standards of nursing care.

This work led to the RCN initiative, Standards of Care Project, which assisted nurses in setting standards as a means of evaluating care. However, before setting standards, nurses needed to participate in a clarification of values exercise.

For the majority of nurses, this was the first time that the values, ideas and beliefs on which their nursing practice was based were seriously considered. They realised that ethics provided the foundation for the attainment of a high standard of nursing care in their own practice. The RCN Society of Paediatric Nursing set up a group to undertake this exercise, of which the editor of this work, Gosia Brykczyńska, was a member. A statement of values was produced and ensuing discussions led to the writing of this much needed book.

In 1983, the United Kingdom Central Council for Nursing, Midwifery and Health Visiting produced its first Code of Professional Conduct (updated 1984). This reminded nurses of their responsibilities and accountability for their practice and the ethics on which professional conduct is founded, and thus further stimulated

Foreword

an interest in the application of nursing ethics to practice.

The editor holds a unique position in paediatric nursing in the United Kingdom, on account of her educational grounding in nursing ethics and her personal interest in relating these to the practice of paediatric nursing. This book will greatly assist paediatric nurses in their ethical thinking and, as the editor states,

concern over ethical issues is not a progressive luxury but an integral part of their (the paediatric nurses') work.

Sue Burr
RCN
November, 1988.

1

Ethics and paediatric nursing practice

GOSIA M. BRYKCZYŃSKA

Nursing has been referred to by some of its practitioners as a moral art and a caring relationship (Tshudin, 1986; Kappeli, 1988); and Curtin categorically states:

Nursing is vitally concerned with ethics because nursing is essentially a moral art, that is, its primary moral conviction shapes its fundamental nature.

(Curtin, 1978).

Certainly from the inception of nursing as a structured professional activity, the ethical components of nursing have been seen as very important, if not central to its practice. Historically however, ethical issues and problems were often seen in a narrow cultural context, so much so, that what was being discussed was etiquette, or cultural norms or legal issues, not ethics as we regard them today (Scrivenger, 1987).

The behaviour of the medieaval abbess administering herbal cures to the indigent sick who came to the abbey for help, was motivated as much by socio-cultural expectations imposed upon her, as by ethical considerations towards the sick (Gies and Gies, 1978). Today's nurses are equally complex in the many motivations they may express that contribute to the quality of their nursing. Ethical reasoning and increased ethical awareness constitute but one aspect of nurses' approach to their work – and yet in another sense 'moral good' should permeate all nursing actions. The influences on moral decisions made by nurses are not any different, however, from those contextual influences that affect the rest of our society. Our nursing lives are fulfilled in a specific historical context, and the philosophical reasoning for our actions will reflect this historical reality.

As we live in a particular time-frame of history, our philosophical understanding and reasoning will be influenced by whatever philosophical theory is most prevalent at the time. Theories of moral philosophy abound as much as other theories pertaining to the structuring and governing of our lives. Although there is overlapping of concepts between the different moral philosophies, they all concern themselves with the nature of good and bad human actions and with the essence of moral behaviour. Enough differences do exist for distinct moral philosophies concerning moral reasoning to have developed, e.g. utilitarianism, Kantian philosophy, existentionalism, etc. These philosophies can be categorized into general areas or approaches to moral reasoning, i.e. theological philosophies or deontological philosophies, but it is beyond the scope of this chapter to analyse the various theories of ethics and explain these differences. Suffice to say that various theories of moral reasoning do exist and we are influenced by them in our thinking to varying degrees. It goes without saying that conscious knowledge of these theories maybe quite meagre or non-existent, e.g. it does not follow that believing in a democratic form of government and majority rule one is cognizant of the philosophical writings of Bentham and Mill, or that belief in fair play means we understand (or indeed have ever read or heard of) the writings of John Rawls. The Judaeo–Christian moral philosophy has strongly influenced the approach of health-care workers to the nature of their work, yet not all health-care workers are Christians or are familiar with the significant writings of that philosophical approach. One can behave according to the rulings of utilitarianism whilst never having understood what utilitarianism is all about. Many people believe in a 'higher authority' or set of rules dictating human conduct and determining the nature of good and bad actions, without ever having heard of deontological reasoning. It is good therefore for thoughtful professionals to study the nature of their reasoning – it can be quite revealing.

Many a nurse will say at this point that she is not consciously aware of having any particular philosophy that underwrites and permeates her approach to life and living. Upon consideration however, with a bit of help from the literature and discussion with peers and friends, most individuals can identify the major source or sources of their moral reasoning. Some individuals refer in their philosophical approaches to an outside authority, e.g. 'I will nurse this patient because of the laws of my God or religion tell me to', others to a combination of cultural and religious norms encompassing several reference points, both external and internal to themselves; and yet others will refer almost exclusively to a non-authoritarian, non-religious humanistic form of reasoning, e.g. an existentionalist approach. As would be expected in a pluralistic society all these forms of reasoning can be identified amongst members of the nursing profession and all members of the nursing profession are influenced in turn by socio-cultural and individual values; so that it is very rare to find someone who demonstrates a pure form of ethical reasoning, straight out of a textbook.

There are many philosophical approaches to life and ways of moral thinking shared by many different people within a specific culture, yet the average practising nurse will not demonstrate an average philosophy, that is, a combination of all philosophies; she will demonstrate an adherence to a particular philosophy, however modified, and carry out her moral reasoning accordingly. It should be fairly clear from this that at any one time, on a ward or in a community setting where several nurses are working, a multiplicity of philosophical approaches may be expressed. In our current socio-political climate we respect varying philosophical approaches, and a multiplicity of philosophies should not be seen as a sign of disarray or disunity of purpose. At the end of the day, all moral reasoning is attempting to guide the moral agent along the most efficacious route to the achievement of maximum goodness. The way in which these philosophies achieve this varies, but at least manifestly the goals remain the same – achieving that which is good.

Just as individuals may be said to have philosophical approaches to life, so professions may be said to develop their own philosophies of practice. As a profession matures and expands and becomes more interactive with the people it serves and works with, it too develops a unique sense of moral reasoning. The nursing profession has been seen to develop socially, e.g. it is now a profession independent of religious constraints, that is, one does not have to lead a monastic or laicized semi-monastic life, as did the early deaconesses in Kaiserworth, in order to pursue a career in nursing. Nursing can be said to have developed culturally and the profession is now seen to be more in touch with the people it serves and works with; thus, the cultural attributes of nursing are seen to be more relevant to the culture in which nurses are practising. For example, in Islamic countries female nurses may wear veils and trousers to work and their employer may be the Green Crescent, whereas their European counterparts may wear tailored dresses with starched caps and work for the Red Cross. The interesting point for us is the extent to which nursing has also been seen to develop morally.

It is the analysis of those nursing concepts categorized as moral values which make up the art and science of the practice of nursing (though they are obviously not exclusive to nursing) that I wish to explore in this chapter.

Some nurses like Curtin, would say we *de facto* are and always were a 'moral' profession, for nursing is

a particularly intense form of general moral commitment (the intensity is directly derivative of the degree of vulnerability of the patient), finding its very roots in the commitment of the nurse–patient relationship.

(Curtin, 1978).

It certainly would appear that we have a heightened awareness of moral issues and ethical decision-making processes, and we are certainly questioning the ethics of our practices (Fry, 1985; Curtin, 1978; Mahon and Fowler, 1979; Dobson, 1986; Lumpp, 1979). We are told by nursing leaders and educationalists to look at our courses for nursing students and include ethics in the new nursing curricula, which are to prepare practitioners for the 1990s and the 21st century (Kileen, 1986; Lanara, 1982; Elsea, 1985; Scrivenger, 1987). It still is not quite clear however, to what extent nursing as a profession has developed morally and to what extent are we examining our practices to determine our professional collective moral accountability. Just as the developing human individual demonstrates healthy growth and maturation by developing morally as well as socio-cognitively and physically, so a profession can be said to show signs of healthy maturational processes when it too starts to develop morally. This may be said to start to occur when the profession begins to question its motivations or, as T.S. Eliot so eloquently stated in *Murder in the Cathedral* (1964), when it starts to examine its so called 'good' actions for their moral status, because

the last temptation is the greatest treason: to do the right deed for the wrong reason.

Perhaps a profession can be said to be truly consolidating its position in society when it starts to reflect on the ethics of its most sacred tenets.

Since a profession, like the profession of nursing, consists of practising individuals who represent conglomerations of biological, cultural, sociological, moral and spiritual norms and values, we can expect the profession to reflect these values also. Just as it is hard to visualize the moral elements in an individual's approach to life, so it may be hard to identify moral strands in the complexity of factors that make a profession in paediatric nursing a holistic entity. Evidence that nursing has moral constituent parts and can be seen to be morally responsive can be demonstrated by analysing the nature of the values held by the nursing profession and transgressing or ignoring any one of them. Since it is quite possible to refer to nursing values (and much has been written of late concerning these values) there must exist concepts corresponding to these values (Thompson, Melia and Boyd, 1983; Steele and Harmon, 1983). If there were no internalized moral values inherent to nursing practice, encompassing all the individual nurses' personal philosophies, then disregarding these nursing values would be of no consequence, certainly of no moral consequence. Indeed we would not even be able to start talking of nursing values at all. Charles Kingsley (1986) expressed this search for the 'known ephemoral' in a delightful way, when he stated that

to prove no water-babies exist, one must see no water-babies existing, which is not the same thing as not seeing water-babies.

The contributors to this book have elaborated upon several values important to the practice of paediatric nursing, but before one can develop the theme of ethical issues one must first define at least one other concept – namely the practice of paediatric nursing.

The practice of paediatric nursing is extremely old, and if one includes non-professional workers, e.g. nannies and wet-nurses, in the historical analysis of the profession, it is indeed a very ancient art and skill. There are several excellent descriptions of the nature of modern professional paediatric nursing, and in 1988 the Association of British Paediatric Nurses celebrated its 50th anniversary as a professional specialist association for paediatric nurses (Burgess, 1988). The areas of work covered by paediatric nursing overlap with all the major paediatric specialities acknowledged by the health-care and medical workers, a selection of which are reflected in this book. It is because paediatric nursing is so diverse that ethical issues can arise, not only inter-professionally but even intra-professionally, and nurses tend to specialize in specific areas of paediatric care and not be very cognizant of problems encountered by their colleagues. The very process of specialization can be seen as generating various ethical questions, for although one of the most common arguments for specialization is increased knowledge about a very circumscribed area, leading to a better quality of care, e.g. renal diseases in childhood, cancer care, school nursing; this high degree of intra-professional specialization inevitably blurs the image of the whole child. Children may be left with an array of attending nursing specialists not one of whom ultimately has total responsibility for the nursing welfare of the child. Perhaps the only solution to this situation is to help prepare the parents for this 'new' role; a role they traditionally have always held and which was taken away from them with the advent of hospital care for children and the emergence of a paternalistic approach towards parents and children in hospitals (Meadow, 1987; Jolly, 1988; Casey, 1988).

Being in a position to control information gives health-care workers considerable power and choice concerning what information is available to whom and at what point in time. This can have significant consequences for the ethical practice of nursing. Historically, medical information was obtained, kept and divulged by physicians – making it essentially a problem of power involving the principle of confidentiality. Nowadays confidentiality binds all health-care workers, and nurses too have to make decisions on such issues as whether they explain in detail to patients about disease processes, when to talk to a nine year old about the potential dangers of treatment non-compliance and are a child's secrets to be kept or can a child's trust be broken? Do we even share our nursing diagnoses and plans with parents? At the heart of these issues lie potential conflicts of principles concerning patient autonomy, confidentiality, veracity and beneficence. Many a parent will suggest that truth be withheld from a child, even though it is a paediatric nursing value always to be truthful to children. In some cases, information transfer may also have legal implications, e.g. in cases of suspected child abuse.

Some children may approach the nurse directly, rather than through another adult, e.g. in the context of a crisis telephone line or during a school physical examination. Information generated during this time may be of far reaching consequences – what of confidentiality now? Fortunately nurses do not work in isolation, and because they have a duty towards the child to share information about him or her with the multidisciplinary childcare team they cannot promise to children or parents that they will never pass on information provided by the patient and his or her family.

Confidentiality does not rule out veracity, and keeping a promise is one of the cardinal principles of ethics – especially when the promise is between two very unequally powerful individuals, such as a child and a nurse.

Giving and receiving information to and from an adolescent poses new problems of confidentiality, veracity and autonomy, which in the main concern the extent to which the adolescent's parents are still involved in parenting. As Lord Fraser pointed out in the summary of the Gillick case in the House of Lords: 'Parental rights to control a child do not exist for the benefit of the parents. They exist for the benefit of the child and they are justified only insofar as they enable the parent to perform his duties towards the child.' If the parents are no longer parenting, to divulge information to them concerning the habits of an adolescent might be an infringement of the adolescent's autonomy and certainly a contravention of the code of confidentiality. It is crucial to understand and assess the level of parental involvement in an adolescent's life. The closer the parents work with and are responsible for the activities of their child, the more important it is that they be given information concerning the child which will help them to parent even better, and that the information gained about the family is kept in confidence to protect the wellbeing of the child and his or her family, who will have to live with the consequences of inaccurate, misplaced or inappropriately divulged information.

It is interesting to note how the concept of care by parents has come full circle and how paediatric nurses have adapted to accommodate this 'new' philosophy (Cheetham, 1988). It is in this climate of change both from within the profession and without that the paediatric nurse must practice her 'moral art'. As Moustakas explains in his therapeutic existentionalist approach to child-care, so the paediatric nurse can echo after him,

As far as it is humanly possible for one person to be in the center of the world of another, I was there, offering myself, my skills, and my strength. It was Jimmy's *experience* that mattered to me.

(Moustakas, 1966).

THE ETHICAL DECISION-MAKING PROCESS

In the course of clinical practice the nurse will undoubtedly come across ethical dilemmas. The extent to which the nurse is aware of ethical issues, that is, has a raised awareness of the existence of potential ethical issues, will determine the frequency with which he or she acknowledges such encounters. Thus, if a nurse perceives administering an incorrect drug solely as a potential cause for a disciplinary hearing, and therefore scrupulously administers the correct drug in order to avoid such a sequence of events, this act will be seen as having no ethical importance to him or her. However, if the nurse avoids giving the incorrect drug because this may harm a patient and cause undue anxiety, then administering the correct drug becomes an ethical issue. The act has become of ethical significance not only because of its inherent value but also because of the value attributed to the action by the nurse. If the incorrect drug was an antacid or a vitamin pill, the nurse on recognizing her error, should she attribute ethical importance to the action, will be faced with an additional complication to the problem. It is this process of recognizing ethical issues and sorting out what to do next that I wish to address in this section.

In bio-ethics one often refers to such deliberations as the ethical decision-making process and essentially what is advocated is a systematic process of analysing data in order to facilitate ethical decision-making. This process may range from a structured sequential analysis of data, to constructing a moral philosophical conceptual framework (Stenberg, 1979). Different practitioners of nursing may consider the significance of nursing issues in diverse ways and attribute quite varying values to them, so that some nurses see very few ethical problems and some see their whole practice effectively based on ethical principles – hence the tensions often felt surrounding some emotive areas. Careful analysis of data that will ultimately justify the decision as being of ethical importance and the analysis of facts surrounding an issue will be a similar practice for all nurses. Phillipa Foot in describing just this issue in terms of evidence for making valid statements said, 'It follows that no two people can make the same statement and count completely different things as evidence, in the end one at least of them could be convicted of linguistic ignorance. It also follows that if a man is given good evidence for a factual conclusion he cannot just refuse to accept the conclusion on the ground that in his scheme of things this evidence is not evidence at all' (Foot, 1967). From such arguments we can see that the more thoroughly an issue is analysed the more likely that the true moral nature of the act will emerge with concensus on whether or not one is looking at an ethical issue of prima facie importance. And so it is that the first step in the process of making an ethical decision is gathering data and determining the nature of known facts.

In the process of gathering information many outside factors will impinge on the values attributed to the facts, and often our own values and philosophical approaches will actually cloud or even alter, quite significantly, what we look for and how we look at a problem. Because of the obvious problems that this can produce, it is beneficial for all the parties involved to be sensitive and aware of their own personal values; a process referred to as 'values clarification'. Such clarification of values is probably very important for permanent senior staff on a ward and an exercise well worth undertaking by all professional nurses whatever the nature of their work. Interesting evaluations of the positive aspects of values clarification and how this can be used effectively by nurses can be readily found among the writings of psychiatric nurses, psychologists and more recently nurse ethicists (Thompson, Melia and Boyd, 1983; Steele and Harman, 1983).

Once information about an issue has been gathered several significant factors will start to emerge. First, at the most basic level of screening it should be possible to ascertain whether or not what is being analysed is of primary ethical importance, for it may well be that it is a social, cultural or even religious problem and not an ethical issue as such. (I avoid here a repetition of the argument that all of our actions at some level have ethical implications, on the assumption that we will take it as given that man is a moral being and nursing is a moral art; but we are not always aware of this and some actions have less obvious ethical implications than others).

It is important to correctly identify the nature of the problem, since to try and tackle the problem as an ethical issue when it is not overtly of moral significance will simply prove unproductive and could itself be seen as ethically questionable. As in all spheres of human activity, the solution must fit the problem; the better the fit, the more likely it is that the problem will be solved.

Another factor that should emerge in the process of collecting data is the extent of existent knowledge concerning a particular case. For example, it is almost impossible to predict satisfactorily treatment outcomes for serious cranial injuries of children injured in road traffic accidents. Some children can make remarkable recoveries from the most extensive trauma, but some will not. The three most significant variables in determining and weighing-up data collected about such a case would be:

1. Is there a body of knowledge describing the treatment outcomes of such children in similar circumstances? This is basically a research approach. The more knowledge there is to back a judgement, the more likely it is that the judgement will be acceptable and valid;

2. What are the local resources available now for the continued treatment of such a child? That is, can the child actually be nursed/cared for – are there the necessary resources? This is a question concerning allocation of resources;

3. What is the expert opinion of the primary health-care providers and parents of the child, concerning probable outcome of continuing treatment under their care? This is a question determining expertise at the local level.

The three points mentioned all involve a degree of knowledge concerning a particular case, and the more information is known the easier it is to make a decision concerning the probable outcome. In the case quoted, which is not uncommon, the extent to which research has described the nature of brain injury and subsequent recovery will profoundly influence any decision. Information about local resources is equally important, for if there are no qualified staff nurses to look after a child, as in a small local hospital, or no moneys available for expensive treatment or diagnostic tests; then several possible moral alternatives will be found impossible to realize in practice. Lastly, the expert opinion of all the health-care providers will not only provide invaluable knowledge concerning the factors already mentioned but also elicit the level of their perceived expertise to deal with such a case. This information, plus the research knowledge and facts concerning resources available, quickly puts into perspective many otherwise seemingly confusing aspects of the case. All problems should be analysed with appropriate questions to help establish a maximum amount of information on which to base one's ethical judgement. To take into account all known facts concerning a case is not only ethically correct, but in fact essential; failure to do so would render whatever solution was finally reached subject to just criticism on the grounds that it represented the result of nothing more than a gut reaction – an automatic response deserving very little serious consideration. Something as important as an ethical decision which is to be acted upon by a multi-disciplinary team should be reached after careful consideration.

There is a type of ethical reasoning (deontological) which argues that one should be solely governed by the laws and principles enshrined in a dictum from an outside authority. For those who subscribe to such reasoning no explanation of their choices is relevant since they argue that they must be doing the 'right thing' if they follow the guidelines imposed upon them. There are some fundamental fallacies in this position; the responsibility for decisions undertaken has been referred to another authority and no question is posed as to the appropriateness of the action in a given situation. We will assume that for the practising nurse aware of his or her professional account-ability and responsibility, full ethical confirmation of decisions will be the norm. The nurse as an intelligent professional will question all that fundamentally affects her work. Curtin addressed the matter well, saying,

A reflective understanding of basic human rights and duties implied by these rights, the ability to weigh possible results of various actions and a considera-tion of situational factors that affect the application of general principles are clearly relevant to accountable nursing practice.

(Curtin, 1978).

The next step in the process is to determine who the ethical agents involved in the particular case are. Often one is confronted with a case where everyone seems to have something to say on the matter but no-one perceives themselves as central to the issue at hand. This can be a crippling situation if a resolution is to be reached, since ultimately someone has to take responsibility for making a decision. Those individuals who are seen as central to an issue or case can be called its ethical agents. Of course, ethical agents may be remote in physical terms but still very important in moral terms, as can be seen in problems of justice and resource allocation where an ethical agent may be a politician or regional health manager. For the most part individuals closely associated with a case can be more readily identi-fied, and in the context of paediatric nursing these must also include the patient and his or her family. All the nurses working with the child and the family (and not just senior nurses, who may be least involved with a case) should be included. It is this group of individuals who will ultimately have some decision to implement and take responsibility for. Sometimes senior managers and senior health-care professionals try to protect junior workers and even family members from the burden of taking responsibility for ethical decisions. Not only is this an illogical practice in an ethical context – for we are all responsible to some extent for the actions of our colleagues and partners-in-care, and this co-responsibility cannot be dismissed easily – but more immediately, it is precisely the junior health-workers and family of a child who bear most heavily the emotional burdens of problematic ethical decisions. They are there with the patient, living and working with the child, at the sharp end of the practice, and to deny them the right and opportunity to make decisions and the psychological value of having an input into an ethical decision-making process, is itself contrary to a healing ethos.

Before any note is taken of moderating factors on any solutions considered – such as what the profession of paediatric nursing has to say on the matter, and what the position of the solution is in law – a list of options can be drawn up. These options can be listed, in the light of identified ethical principles that the ethical agents have singled out as problematic. The identification of these principles and/or rules will be largely determined by the philosophical biases of the ethical agents; but on the whole one can state that identifying principles of ethical behaviour helps in clarifying the issue that is being analysed. Often one hears from nurses, 'but honestly there is/was nothing else we could do'. Although superficially this may seem to be the case, every human action has an alternative action that can replace it. Not all of these will turn out to be sensible, logical, safe, legal or culturally acceptable, but they are all alternative modes of action. Unless one can identify what these alternative actions may be, it becomes futile to discuss an ethical decision-making process. Making a decision implies the use of a logical sequential thought process in the selection of a particular choice of action from a range of alternatives. If no alternative forms of action are identified then one cannot talk of choices in decision-making. It should now become clearer why one should spend such a proportionally large amount of time and energy on collecting information about a case.

Identifying potential alternative actions is not always easy, e.g. in the case of a child with end-stage osteogenic sarcoma that has proven non-responsive to traditional medical treatment, it may be futile to continue with established therapies; however, unless alternative treatments to this course of traditional therapy are identified by the ethical agents it may be difficult to change the current course of ineffective treatments. The alternatives for the child may range from complete withdrawal of medical intervention except for symptom control, to homeopathic remedies, folk-remedies, experimental medicine or even some form of religious intervention. If we had research evidence that the folk-remedy was not therapeutic then it could not be seriously considered for implementation as this would be contrary to an ethical approach, according to the principle of Beneficence. However, an even more interesting ethical dilemma could ensue if the recommended folk-remedy was seen to be efficacious occasionally. The listing and then systematic refutation of arguments is another aid to help clarify the thought processes, and one often used by moral philosophers.

Several assumptions have been made here, most notably that all the ethical agents involved are articulate and skilled communicators. Although this is patently not always the case, in this context it is important to remember that inarticulation and uncertainty is a personal characteristic of immense importance and to be taken into consideration. No one of the ethical agents should have a more important voice in the discussion just because of training, education or social class. All should be equal partners in the decision-making; it will often be the child and its family, if anyone, who carry greatest responsibility overall, therefore great weight should be attributed to what they say, however 'unprofessionally' they say it.

The course of action decided upon ought to reflect the resolution of conflict or dilemma resulting from identified conflicting ethical claims. The professional ethical agents need also to bear in mind what their respective professional bodies might have to say concerning the decision that is being considered. The study of the code of professional conduct (UKCC, 1984) is a last chance for the nurse to determine the ethical nature of her professional conduct. Thus, a nurse may have reached the decision that it is unethical to continue administering intramuscular injections of an antibiotic to a toddler every four hours, and that an alternative administration route ought to be found. She may now verify the acceptability of this decision by consulting the code of professional conduct, the hospitals' philosophy of nursing, the charter of children's rights and the district policies. Hopefully, the points in the code of professional conduct will have been sufficiently internalized by the nurse that she is quite aware of the spirit of the code and its content. The nurse is well read in aspects of pain control and pain theory in children, in keeping with the recommendation of the code to maintain professional competence, and her understanding of accountability leads her to take on an interventionalist position *vis-à-vis* with another colleague's orders for child-care. A very large percentage of nurses' ethical problems are generated extra-professionally. Fortunately for the nurse, the current philosophy of paediatric nursing supports and encourages an empathetic approach to nursing children. If the nurse was uncertain what to do however, consultation with a relevant senior person in the nursing profession would be called for, i.e. a senior paediatric nurse. It is important to verify the professional acceptability of an action before it is enacted, not only to ascertain the intrinsic value of the proposed alternative solution, but also because the patient relationship demands the best we have to offer, and this includes consultation with our peers over our professional accountability. Sister Lumpp, in describing the role of the nurse in the bio-ethical decision-making process, identifies reverence and fidelity as the two components of the advocacy relationship (Lumpp, 1979). In order to keep these qualities intact, it is important to ensure that decisions are made with as wide a consultation as possible, so that what is being instituted does not become just a personal solution. Finally, a decision once enacted is sometimes hard or impossible to reverse, so for all concerned it is better to consult with other professional colleagues first.

There is, in conclusion, one final moderating force that has to be considered by all citizens of the land, and that is the legal implications of an action. Local hospitals or area health authorities may have procedural policies and/or guidelines to which all employees are bound and should be familiar with. Although these policies may not always have the full power of law, they govern practice locally and any transgressions should be made extremely cautiously. If a particular policy turns out to be unmanageable or impractical then it is the responsibility of the practitioners governed by this policy to attempt to have it altered so that it is possible to be practising intelligently within the guidelines of the policies. It is good to remember here that laws of the land, for the most part, adhere to universal principles of ethics, especially the concepts of justice and non-malevolence, but the particular interpretation of the law in a specific case can sometimes result in a conflict of the law with personal philosophy. The law, by definition, must be universally applicable, and it is professionals and patients who must measure their behaviour against the law (Scrivenger, 1987). Responsibility for acting illegally cannot be abolished by reference to ethical motivations for breaking the law in the first place. Ethical motivation may help diminish a subsequent penalty for illegal behaviour but it cannot remove legal responsibility for the action.

In some parts of the world governments have attempted to legislate on certain aspects of bio-ethical decision-making, which in turn can pose ethical dilemmas for health-care practitioners working within the constraints of the law. This has been most clearly demonstrated in the USA, where it was legislated that all neonates be actively treated irrespective of other chronic conditions that might be present. Research into such areas of nursing concern is very interesting; Savage's study illustrates (Savage, Cullen, Kirchoff, 1987) that this puts nurses under enormous strain and adds to their already high stress levels. It somehow is not fair, as Curtin pointed out, that in the pursuance of one's job it is necessary to practice heroic virtue (Curtin, 1978). Fowler, in a recent article, poignantly pointed out that to nurse under such conditions calls for more than average sensibilities – quoting Robb who almost a century ago was advocating that nurses be 'intelligent saints' (Fowler, 1986).

Every child should have the opportunity to be treated, and to undergo corrective surgery, especially if this is life-restoring. The problem is not in a rejection of the principle of justice (equal opportunities and access to treatment for all children) but with the idea that just because something can be done, it should be done. What in fact are the limits of technological and medical interventions? The realization in practice of such an approach to health-care is equally unethical as it disregards the ethical concepts of the rights of the patient and family to make autonomous decisions. Sometimes for a neonate to die is quite natural and normal if it has a combination of congenital defects such that the child is incapable of sustaining its fragile hold on life. Inflicting unjustifiable pain and suffering on a child (and there is an ever increasing wealth of knowledge concerning paediatric pain) who deserves more respect than to be the anonymous recipient of a blanket approach to medical and surgical prowess is hard to explain away in moral terms. This common problem in neonatology does not refer, however, to those cases of instituting a single life-promoting act or life-saving procedure, whether performed as a single permanent intervention, or in order to give health-care workers time to think about subsequent interventions, e.g. in the case of correcting duodenal atresia in newborns with Down's syndrome, closing the open back of a child with myelomeningocele, or implanting a ventriculoperitoneal shunt for a child with idiopathic hydrocephalus. In all such cases the background information, scrupulously gathered at the beginning of the process, all determine the nature of the decision undertaken, a point often stressed in the Zachary-Lorber debate over the selective non-treatment of children with myelomeningocele (Weir, 1984). Potential political or legal interference in ethical decisions, by the imposition of universally binding legal constraints, can be counter-productive, if protecting the rights and dignity of individual children is what the law is attempting to promote. Some multiply-handicapped children should be cared for without drastic medical interventions if in fact they are incapable of sustaining life. Inflicting pain in the form of medical and surgical treatment can only be justified if it promotes a reasonable quality of life, restores life or measurably increases the child's potential to live a normal life.

Many a multiply-handicapped youngster *is* an appropriate surgical candidate for corrective interventions where surgery can improve or enhance gait, speech, vision, hearing and so on. However, when these interventions are carried out primarily for social or cosmetic reasons some parents may object to the underlying motivation for the surgery.

The second point to bear in mind is the position of the law regarding nursing interventions which are seen to be ethical but might be illegal. Since we must always act ethically and, given choices of action, always choose that action which most closely approaches a perfect moral solution, sometimes to do that which one considers morally correct may conflict with what is allowed by law. Sometimes the conflict arises because of the nature of the philosophical theory to which one subscribes (often in the form of deontological reasoning), where even though some therapeutic intervention is possible it is not a considered alternative for the ethical agent, as would be the case in blood transfusing for a Jehovah's Witness, limb amputation for some religious groups and, increasingly, organ transplantations for many others. Parents may dearly love their children and wish that which is best for them, but some therapeutic options are just not negotiable for such parents (or indeed nurses, either). Intervention by the law may or may not save the life of the child, but it certainly violates several ethical principles in respect of the parent. Often decisions are taken before a thorough investigation of the case, when looking intelligently and in a dispassionate manner at a problematic case could throw light on alternative solutions which are more acceptable to all the ethical agents involved. There is, of course, little need to discuss cases of conflict in which an action is considered unethical but otherwise legal, as from the position of the law no repercussions can occur, although it is as well to understand the distinction between legality of an action and its ethical merits.

Now the nurse can start to implement the ethical decision that she has reached. As the decision is undertaken it is monitored and effects of the decision are carefully noted. In some cases additional intervention might be required with new appraisals, and if the situation changes sufficiently then a new ethical decision-making process might have to be instituted.

An example of just such a process was seen in the events following the decision to discontinue artificial ventilation of Karen Quinlan who was presumed irretrievably brain damaged in permanent coma, surviving solely with the aid of artificial ventilation (Lamb, 1985). When she was removed from the ventilator she started to breathe spontaneously and a new decision had to be undertaken to support her fragile life until she died naturally, which turned out to be for another twelve years. Ethical decision-making can therefore be seen to be cyclical in nature.

Nurses often say, 'I know I did the right thing because I felt good about it afterwards'. There are some problems with such an argument; the most elemental being that this is not a universal criteria for assessing the moral good of an action. Take for example the case of discontinuing medical treatment for severely neurologically impaired neonates. The decision may well be ethically sound, since medical science has nothing to offer this child that will change the diagnosis or prognosis, and it is not reasonable to expend disproportionate amounts of time and energy to prolong an inevitable dying process in a painful and distressing manner for the child. The decision once undertaken, may mean that nurses who understand the rationale for the decision undertaken will still have to nurse this infant with love and care until it dies, which can be varying lengths of time. The distress of nurses as they work through their own, and the family's, anticipatory grief may be very high, and they may feel very ambivalent about the decision; but ultimately, since it is a shared decision of all ethical agents, the nursing care of the child is sensitive to and supportive of the basic needs of the child and the family. In retrospect the nurses will be able to conclude that they did not like having to watch the child die. It did not feel 'good', or 'right', but at least they nursed him or her faithfully until her death. They maintained the covenant relationship, and stood in reverential awe of the dignity of the patient (Lumpp, 1979). There have been cases where severely neurologically impaired children, e.g. microcephalic infants, have been abandoned in hospitals and left to die without the overt love and care of their families. When it came to arranging the funeral it was nurses on the unit who attended the service and accompanied the coffin to the grave-side – they had, for a short time, stood in for the family. Undertaking difficult decisions does not therefore necessarily make one feel 'good' or 'bad'. The sole criteria for knowing that a positive moral decision was taken at the time, is the certainty that all possible options were looked at, analysed and measured up to identified ethical principles. In the end, one cannot do more than that which is seen as the best decision at the time.

The nurse may feel at this point that the bio-ethical decision-making process is elaborate and impractical and one which could never be implemented 'on my ward'. Luckily, for overworked staff nurses, as professional expertise grows, so the process of making decisions becomes easier and takes less time. A lot of the preparatory work that goes into making a decision is in fact an ongoing process of personal maturation and ethical consciousness raising. Collective wisdom is important and the sharing of knowledge, experiences and attitudinal differences can become excellent avenues of experimential learning – hence the enormous benefit of 'clarifying values'. The more nurses communicate with each other and other health-care workers, the less stressful incidences there will be and the less extraneous tension on the wards and in the workplace. Ethical decision-making can then take place in an environment of mutual trust and respect (a quality not just reserved for patients, but governing all health-care workers). Incidently, better inter-professional communications may help cut down some of the ethical issues arising from role misconceptions and institutional paternalism (Wilson-Barnett, 1986). Finally paediatric nurses care about children, and in the pursuit of an ever better quality of care for the children, they have an obligation to develop morally. If nurses take too long to respond to moral problems and reach moral maturity then it may be too late for them to help their young patients, because

this thing is sure, that time is no healer: the patient is no longer here.

(Eliot, 1963).

Paediatric nurses must be constantly raising their ethical awareness and be open and willing to change when and if necessary. They must learn to be empathetic. If they start looking at their care of children with a child's eye, in a child's manner, and see their obligations towards the child and its family as a responsibility of love, then the 'burden' of their work will become more bearable also. If the child 'suffers unbearably' (Evely, 1967) in its process of socialization to adulthood, nurses too should strive to recall that process. In conclusion, the nurse, like Martin Buber, should strive to identify wholly with the child: that should be the paediatric nurse's basis of all his or her ethical reasoning for,

in order to be and remain truly present to the child he must have gathered the child's presence into his own store as one of the bearers of his communion with the world, one of the focuses of his responsibilities for the world . . . If he has really gathered the child into his life then that subterranean dialogic, that steady potential presence of the one to the other is established and endures. Then there is reality between them, there is mutuality.

(Buber, 1947).

REFERENCES

Buber, M. (1947) in *Between Man and Man*. Routledge and Kegan Paul, London, p.98.

Burgess, T. (1988) No more potty rounds. *Nursing Times*, **84** (16) 69–71.

Casey, A. (1988) A partnership with child and family. *Senior Nurse*, **8** (4) 8–9.

Cheetham, T. (1988) Model care in the surgical ward. *Senior Nurse*, **8** (4) 10–12.

Curtin, L.L. (1978) Nursing ethics: theories and pragmatics. *Nursing Forum*, **17** (1) 4–11.

Dobson, S. (1986) Cultural value awareness: glimpse into a Punjabi mother's world. *Health Visitor*, **59** (12) 382–4.

Eliot, T.S. (1963) *Collected Poems 1909–1962*. Faber and Faber, London.

Eliot, T.S. (1964) *Murder in the Cathedral*. Harcourt Brace and Jovanovich, London.

Elsea, S.B. (1985) Ethics in maternal-child nursing. *MCN* **10** (5) 303–8.

Evely, L. (1967) *Suffering*. Herder and Herder, New York.

Foot, P. (1967) *Theories of Ethics*. Oxford University Press, Oxford.

Fowler, M.D. (1986) Ethics without virtue. *Heart and Lung* **15** (5) 528–30.

Fry, S.T. (1985) Individual vs aggregate good: ethical tension in nursing pratice. *Int. J. Nurs. Studies*, **22** (4), 303–10.

Gies, F. and Gies, J. (1978) *Women in the Middle Ages*. Barnes and Noble Books, New York.

Jolly, J. (1988) Meeting special needs of children in hospital. *Senior Nurse*, **8** (4) 6–7.

Kappeli, S. (1988) *To build anew – but what about the patient*. Paper presented at the Royal College of Nursing Annual Research Society Conference, April 1988, Belfast.

Kileen, M.L. (1986) Nursing fundamental texts: where's the ethics? *J. Nurs. Educ.*, **25** (8) 334–9.

Kingsley, C. (1986) *The Water Babies*. Puffin Classics, Penguin, Harmondsworth, Middx.

Lamb, D. (1985) *Death, Brain Death and Ethics*. Croom Helm, London.

Lanara, A.V. (1982) Responsibility in nursing. *Int. Nurs. Rev.*, **29** (1) 7–10.

Lumpp, F. (1979) The role of the nurse in the bio-ethical decision making process. *Nursing Clinics of North America*, **14** (1) 13–21.

Mahon, K.A. and Fowler, M.D. (1979) Moral development and clinical decision making. *Nursing Clinics of North America*, **14** (1), 3–12.

Meadow, R. (1987) Children's Services The Problems and Prospects of Rationalisation Cost and Quality in Child Health, Conference, King's Fund Centre, London.

Moustakas, Clark (ed.) (1966) *The Child's Discovery of Himself, Introduction – The Existential Moment*. Ballantine Books, New York.

Savage, T.A., Cullen, D.L., Kirchhoff, K.T., Pugh, E.T. and Foreman, D.M. (1987) Nurses responses to DNR–NICU. *Nursing Research*, **36** (6).

Scrivenger, M. (1987) Ethics, etiquette and the law. *Nursing Times*, **83** (42) 28–9.

Steele, S. and Harmon, V. (1983) *Values Clarification in Nursing*. 2nd edn, Appleton-Century-Croft, New York.

Stenberg, M.J. (1979) The Search for a Conceptual Framework as a Philosophic Basis for Nursing Ethics: An Examination of Code, Contract, Context and Covenant Military Medicine. **144** (1), 9–21.

Thompson, I.E., Melia, K.M. and Boyd, K.M. (1983) *Nursing Ethics*. Churchill Livingstone, Edinburgh.

Tshudin, V. (1986) *Ethics in Nursing: The Caring Relationship*. Heineman Nursing, London.

UKCC (1984) *United Kingdom Central Council Code of Professional Conduct for the Nurse, Midwife and Health Visitor*. 2nd edn, UKCC, London.

Weir, R. (1984) *Selective Non-treatment of Handicapped Newborns*. Oxford University Press, Oxford.

Wilson–Barnett, J. (1986) Ethical dilemmas in nursing. *J. Med. Ethics*, **12** (3) 123–6.

FURTHER READING

Ackerman, T.F. (August, 1980) *The Limits of Beneficence, Jehovah's Witnesses and Childhood Cancer.* The Hastings Center Report, Hastings-on-Hudson, NY.

Anderson, S. (1975) A child's view of a pediatric bill of rights. *Pediatr,* 55 (3) p 370.

Atchison, N. *et al* (1986) Pain in the pediatric burn patient: nursing assessment and perception. *Issues in Comprehensive Pediatric Nursing,* 9, pp 399–409.

Beauchamp, T.L. and Childress, J.F. (1983) *Principles of Biomedical Ethics.* 2nd edn, Oxford University Press, Oxford.

Benjamin, P. and Curtis, S. (1986) *Ethics in Nursing* (2nd edn), Oxford University Press, Oxford.

Burr, S. (1987) *Quality of Care – is it measurable?* Cost and Quality in Child Health, Conference held at King's Fund Centre, London.

Chaney, E.A. (1986) The rights of disabled infants. *J. Pediatr. Nurs.,* 1 (6) pp 409–11.

Cherry, B.S. and Carty, R.M. (1986) Changing concepts of childhood in society. *Pediatr. Nurs.,* 12 (6) pp 779–87.

Davis, A.J. and Aroskar, M.A. (1983) *Ethical Dilemmas and Nursing Practice.* 2nd edn, Appleton-Century-Crofts, NY.

Drane, J.F. (1984) The defective child: ethical guidelines for painful dilemmas. *JOGN Nursing,* 13 (1), 42–8.

Dyer, C. (1985) The Gillick Judgement, Contraceptives and the under 16's: House of Lords Ruling. *Br. Med. J.,* 291 (6503) 1208–9.

Eland, J.M. and Anderson, J.E. (1977) The experience of pain in children. In Jacox, A.K. (ed.) *Pain: a sourcebook for nurses and other health professionals.* Little Brown, Boston, pp 453–73.

Felton, G.M. and Parson, M.A. (1987) The impact of nursing education on ethical/moral decision making. *J. Nurse Educ.,* 26 (7), pp 7–11.

Fotion, N.G. (1985) Ethics and the Afflicted Child, Critical Care Quarterly. 8 (3) pp 75–82.

Franck, L.S. (1986) A new method of qualitatively describing pain behaviour in infants. *Nursing Research,* 35, pp 28–31.

Frankenna, W.K. (1973) *Ethics.* Prentice Hall Inc., Englewood Cliffs, NY.

Gadow, S. (1980) Existential advocacy: a philosophical foundation of nursing. In Spicker, S.F. and Gadow, S. (eds) *Nursing: Images and Ideals,* Springer, NY.

Gramelspacher, G.P., Howell, J.D. and Young, M.J. (1986) Perception of ethical problems by nurses and doctors. *Arch. Intern. Med.,* 146 (3), pp 577–8.

Jolly, H. (1984) Have parents the right to see their children's medical reports? *Arch. Dis. Child.,* 59, (7), pp 601–2.

Mause de Lloyd, (ed.) (1974) *The History of Childhood*. Harper and Row, NY.

Mill, J.S. (1958) *Utilitarianism*. Liberal Arts Press, New York.

Murphy, C. (1976) Making ethical decisions systematically. *Nursing*, 76, pp 13–15.

Owens, M.E. and Todt, E.H. (1984) Pain in infancy: neonatal response to heel lance. *Pain*, 20, pp 77–86.

Pinch, W.J. (1985) Ethical dilemmas in nursing: the role of the nurse and perceptions of autonomy. *J. Nurs. Educ.*, 24 (9), pp 372–6.

Pyne, R. (1981) *Professional Discipline in Nursing, Theory and Practice*. Blackwell Scientific Publications, Oxford.

Pyne, R. (1987) A professional duty to shout. *Nursing Times*, 83 (42), pp 30–1.

Rawls, J. (1971) *The Theory of Justice*. Harvard University Press, Cambridge, Massachusetts.

Verzemnieks, I. and Nash, D. (1984) Ethical issues related to paediatric care. *Nursing Clinics of North America*, 19 (2), pp 319–28.

Webb, N., Hull, D., Madeley, R. (1985) Care by parents in hospital. *Br. Med. J (Clin. Res.)*, 291, 176–7.

2

Ethics in neonatal nursing

DOROTHY A. WHYTE

The power of modern technology to save the lives of infants who would previously have perished evokes a response of admiration and wonder when the result is successful, but something nearer anguish and recrimination when the outcome is less favourable.

The long-term results of intensive care for infants of low birth-weight are on the whole encouraging. In one centre, between 1981 and 1986, 88% of infants weighing less than 1500 g survived to go home, and it was expected that 90% of survivors would be able to go to a normal school (McIntosh, 1987). Surgical repair of congenital cardiac anomalies is currently in the news because the demand has outstripped resources, particularly of paediatric nurses trained in intensive care. Other handicapping conditions have incurred a different response, and we shall examine the dilemmas which are presented when a neonate with a neurological defect requires surgery for a further abnormality. In this chapter I shall discuss trends in medical treatment of the severely handicapped newborn, with reference to the complex legal and ethical issues involved. The interests of the child, the family and society will be considered. Finally the dilemmas will be analysed in relation to nursing practice.

The dilemmas are not new. In more primitive cultures and in the fragile economies of Third World countries strenuous efforts to save the lives of severely handicapped newborn infants are rare. From my memories of nurse training thirty years ago in Britain, before surgical intervention for spina bifida and hydrocephalus had advanced, medical orders were given to withhold feeding from badly damaged infants. The absurd and tragic situation of night nurses surreptitiously feeding starving infants was not uncommon. Such situations however did not attract media attention and were not open to debate.

TRENDS IN TREATMENT

Probably the first neonatologists to report deaths associated with discontinuance or withdrawal of treatment were Duff and Campbell (1973), working at Yale University. Forty three deaths over a 2½ year period were in this category, and examples were given of the nature of the handicapping conditions and the decisions taken. One was an infant with Down's syndrome and intestinal atresia, who was not treated because his parents thought that surgery was wrong for their baby and for themselves. The medical management and nursing care is not discussed, but the child died seven days after birth. Attempts to rescue another infant persisted for five months, following severe idiopathic respiratory distress syndrome requiring positive pressure ventilation with high concentrations of oxygen. When oxygen supplementation was finally stopped the baby died within three hours. The strain undergone by the infant's parents was a contributing factor to the decision reached. The writers take a compassionate stance and clearly spent considerable time with parents to help them to understand the prognosis and share in the decision-making. They readily acknowledged the dangers of an 'allocation of death' policy but argued that the uncontrolled application of medical technology may be detrimental to individuals and to families.

In a more recent study entitled *Death as an option in neonatal intensive care*, Whitelaw (1986) reported on withdrawal of treatment over a four year period in the regional neonatal intensive care unit at Hammersmith Hospital, London. The criterion for non-treatment or withdrawal of treatment was near-certainty of death or no meaningful life. Seventy five infants had their treatment reviewed under this criterion; 26 had severe acquired neurological damage, 26 were born after a gestation period of 25 weeks or less, and 23 had severe congenital abnormalities. The decision to withdraw treatment had to be unanimous among all the medical and nursing staff involved, and was based on a virtual certainty of total incapacity, e.g. microcephaly, spastic quadriplegia and blindness. The decision of the medical team was to withdraw treatment from 51 of the 75 infants. The decisions were fully discussed with the parents, reviewing the whole medical history, the infant's current status and likely prognosis.

It was then suggested to the parents that the intensive care was not restoring health but merely prolonging an uncomfortable life or postponing death. Since the treatment was ineffective, the medical decision was to stop treatment. There was then a pause for the parents' reactions. If the parents indicated that they understood and accepted the medical assessment, treatment was stopped and the parents were encouraged to hold the infant in their arms. If the parents could not accept the medical conclusion and did not want support withdrawn, treatment was continued. Further assessment and discussion could take place later.

The parents of four infants chose to continue intensive care, and two of these infants survived, though with disabilities. The parents of the remaining 47 seriously ill neonates accepted the medical decision and all these infants died. It is not clear from the paper what kind of terminal care these infants received or how long it took them to die. Whitelaw clearly felt that some of the children in the group of 75 who were considered for withdrawal of treatment but were reprieved, would have been better not to have survived due to their 'pathetic and joyless existence' and the strain they imposed on the rest of the family.

These papers bring into the open dilemmas which the public would rather not know about. The writers have been prepared to lay their management decisions before their colleagues and invite debate. In both situations it was emphasized that the decisions were made by consensus and the parents involved in decision-making, though not left with the responsibility for it. Whitelaw stated that if the decision was not unanimous within the medical and nursing team, treatment was continued.

To stop treatment, when it resulted in the death of an infant, was an irrevocable step, whereas if treatment were continued the infant could be reassessed later.

A contrast is made between the 1973 study in Yale, in which 14% of neonatal deaths followed withdrawal of treatment, and the 30% in Hammersmith, in which extremely short gestation or severe acquired neurological damage were the causes of death, rather than congenital defects. Within Duff and Campbell's report was an infant with Down's syndrome and intestinal atresia. Whitelaw would not have considered this sufficient grounds for withdrawal of treatment, since children with such a disorder can still lead happy and active lives.

Looking at the data it is hard to disagree with the decision to bring to a humane end these unfortunate lives. There are, however, issues which require further examination before a pragmatic approach can be accepted.

Probably the first openly pragmatic approach to such questions in Britain was that advocated by Lorber, a paediatric surgeon who, in the seventies, became so concerned about the outcome of surgical repair of myelomeningocele that he advocated the use of selection criteria to exclude the more severely affected infants from surgical intervention (Lorber, 1974). There was some media coverage of the issue at that time; an interesting point which emerged during a television documentary was the powerful influence of medical advice on the parents' decision-making. Two surgeons who took diametrically opposed stands on the issue of non-treatment could show that, having discussed each individual case fully with parents, they would offer a second opinion, which was invariably refused and the doctor's advice accepted. This would seem to give support to the current practice of open discussion with parents while protecting them from the whole burden of decision-making, but it also places a heavy responsibility on medical staff to examine their own motives, attitudes and knowledge base in reaching difficult decisions. The fact is that the principle of selection has been largely adopted in relation to surgery for myelomeningocele, although the subject is still open to discussion (Rosenbloom and Cudmore, 1985).

Too often, however, the discussion is in medical journals while public opinion is neither explored nor expressed.

MEDICO–LEGAL ISSUES

These issues attract public debate when an individual case becomes the centre of legal action. The best known of these in Britain was the Arthur case in 1981. John P. was born with Down's syndrome in June, 1980. The late Dr Leonard Arthur was the consultant paediatrician and he wrote in the case notes 'Parents do not wish it to survive. Nursing care only'. He then prescribed sedation, and the baby died of 'bronchopneumonia due to the consequences of Down's syndrome' 69 hours after birth (Shearer, 1984). A member of the organization Life informed the police and in February 1981 Dr Arthur was charged with murder. He denied the charge.

It was found on post-mortem that baby John had had some

damage to heart, lungs and brain as well, but this was not known at the time the life-terminating decision was taken. It gave the defence grounds, however, to claim that the prosecution case had been conceived in ignorance and inaccuracy. The judge directed that the charge should be changed to attempted murder and the jury acquitted Dr Arthur of the charge.

The medical profession largely gave its support to Dr Arthur. The press was divided, as was public opinion. The report prepared by Shearer for the Campaign for Mentally Handicapped People gives a helpful summary of the press response at that time.

The Times was fairly clear: Every live-born baby enters civil society and by doing so acquires independent rights, of which the chief concerns life itself. He is no less entitled than the rest of us to receive all available life support, save only in those grave and exceptional cases where he lacks irremediably the capacity to live a recognizably human life.

The Guardian was less sure: An area as complex as this one cannot be reduced to formulae, to a consistent pattern . . . Just as the slippery slope argument shouldn't be used to bind doctors to an absolute of survival, so it should not be used to allow them to kill. Just as the law is necessary to ensure that doctors observe these boundaries, so it should not be abused by fanatical absolutionists (*sic*) who wish to undermine a doctor's freedom to act in his patients' best interests.

The divided opinion of society was demonstrated by a MORI poll commissioned by the Human Rights Society in 1982. The question was put:

When parents feel that they cannot cope with a severely handicapped newborn baby should it be arranged
(a) for the baby to die by withholding food or necessary medical treatment
(b) for the baby to be looked after in a home or hospital for the handi- capped or by foster parents?

Thirty seven per cent of respondents chose the first of the alter- natives, 45% the second, 13% were undecided and 5% gave a different reply. (*The Times*, 26.3.82.)

In the United States at this time the issues concerning the handicapped newborn were given a high profile by the involvement of the government. Baby Doe was born in Indiana in 1982 with Down's syndrome and oesophageal atresia with tracheo–oesophageal fistula. The obstetrician said that he would be severely retarded – a prediction that could not have been made with any accuracy at that stage – and that the mortality rate for the surgical procedure to correct the oesophageal atresia was 50%. It is doubtful if many paediatric surgeons would admit to such a high mortality rate for this type of surgical repair. Indeed the paediatrician involved in this case thought that the infant should be referred for surgical treatment but the parents accepted the obstetrician's advice and refused consent for surgery.

The following day the obstetrician ordered the infant to be fed but told the nurses that this would result in the baby choking to death (Koop, 1987a). The intensive care nurses revolted and the baby had to be transferred to a private room and was given phenobarbitol and morphine. Lawyers sought a court order for intravenous feeding which was refused. The infant died in the midst of a controversy which opened the way for changes in legislation.

In 1983 the Department of Health and Human Services (DHHS) at President Reagan's directive, issued an interim ruling relating the 1973 Rehabilitation Act to the care of handicapped newborns. This included posting signs in specific patient care areas affirming the right to feeding and customary medical care of all handicapped infants, and providing a hotline for anonymous callers to report suspected violations. While this move had the support of the Pro-Life campaigners and such organizations as the Association for Retarded Citizens, it ran into fierce opposition from medical organizations (Shearer, 1984). Following heated public debate and prolonged controversy between professional groups and government bodies the ruling was withdrawn and Congress enacted amendments to child abuse legislation which gave protection to handicapped infants. There were interpretive guidelines clarifying the legal position. Treatments defined as futile or prolonging the act of dying of a terminally ill infant were not required. Everett Koop, who was Surgeon–General of the Public Health Service at that time, and himself a paediatric surgeon, commented, 'In spite of the apparent deference to reasonable medical judgement there was underlined in the regulations a presumption in favour of treatment.'

It can be argued that direction of medical practice through government legislation is not the ideal way to resolve ethical dilemmas, although it is to be hoped that a moral consensus will ultimately give legal sanction to good practice. In what direction is the moral consensus going, or indeed, is there any consensus? What factors influence people's thinking about these problems?

SOCIAL IMPLICATIONS

A New York newspaper ran a series of articles in 1984 on 'Human issues of high-tech medicine' which examined individual cases of handicap and prematurity within a wider context of the emotional and financial cost to parents, and the responsibility of doctors and of society (Colen and Kerr, 1984). There was clear concern about the ill-considered application of technology, particularly in relation to very low birth-weight infants. The picture painted, however, did give a bleak impression of the outcome of technological support. It was stated that an ever-growing number of pre-term infants who had received life-saving treatment at birth were growing into young children who could be called prisoners of technology, their lungs being so damaged by disease and the machines used to save them that they could not be removed from the machines. The individual examples given were all of infants who were to some extent brain damaged as a result of treatment. The writers were trying to help society as a whole 'to confront its own painful decisions, on allocation of medical resources and application of medical technology'. The resource allocation problem has greater personal impact in the United States, although federal and state governments do now share responsibility for the nation's hospital bills. In the current political and economic climate in the UK, where value for money is something of a watchword, the expense of technical support for infants 'on the edge of viability' (Colen and Kerr, 1984) may well be questioned. Garland (1983) looked at studies which examined the resource allocation issue. One of these costed rescue efforts for infants 1000 g or less at birth and deemed the expense justified because the overall survival rate had improved, and at that time 70% of survivors were developmentally normal (Pomerance *et al*, 1978). Another study by Shannon *et al* (1981) found that intensive care for infants, per patient was 52% less costly than for adults, that the infants had a 43% greater likelihood of survival than adults, and that there was a much greater probability of normal productive life for the infant survivors as compared with adult survivors. The writers of the most comprehensive study judged that neonatal intensive care was markedly cost-effective for infants about 1000 g birth-weight threshold (Budetti *et al*, 1981). Below that threshold there appeared to be an increased chance that a severely abnormal infant would survive as a result of intensive care. The conclusion was, however, that the increased number of normal and near-normal survivors in the above 1000 g birth-weight group would offset, for policy purposes, the excess costs associated with an increase in the rate of severely abnormal survivors.

It is unlikely that the argument for withdrawal of treatment would be made on the grounds of financial cost alone, but it is helpful to be aware of the economic facts when reference is so often made to the financial burden caused by unsuccessful intensive care.

ETHICAL QUESTIONS

Having looked at some of the medical, legal and economic aspects of the treatment of handicapped newborns there remain ethical issues to be examined. Questions at the heart of the matter are:

Should every effort be made to save every human life?
Are some lives of more value than others?
Can a decision for non-treatment be compatible with the values of justice, beneficence and respect for persons?
Which considerations should bear most weight in the decision-making process – the child's right to life, the family's capacity to cope, or the burden on society?

We cannot hope to arrive at answers to all these very difficult questions, but we can examine arguments and positions, and attempt to identify principles which will guide practice.

The values of justice, i.e. of equal rights; of beneficence, i.e. seeking the good of others, and respect for persons, i.e. seeing each person as an individual of infinite worth, have underpinned western society for well over 2000 years. They are part of our Judaeo–Christian heritage. In his consideration of cultural influences on ethical decision-making, Rumbold (1986) shows that while medical intervention on behalf of severely handicapped infants may not be required in such major world religions as Islam and Hinduism, or in some branches of the Christian church, active euthanasia of the handicapped newborn would be proscribed by all. Only in Marxism, where a doctor's duty is to the State rather than to the individual, could a decision to end an infant's life be considered justified on the grounds that survival would place an unnecessary strain on society's resources.

The widely held ideas of right and wrong, of human rights and freedoms, are not confined to particular religious beliefs, but are underpinned by what has been described as natural law. It is argued that, rather as there are natural laws governing the physical universe, so there are natural laws governing human behaviour and decision making. They provide a foundation for moral statements and ethical codes. The way in which they are applied to the solving of ethical dilemmas, however, varies considerably, and by the very nature of these hard choices it is difficult, if not impossible, to meet the best interests of all involved. Also in recent years arguments have been developed which call into question values which have previously been considered absolute.

Kuhse and Singer (1985) claim that even those who defend the view that all human life is of equal worth do not in fact take the rhetoric seriously. They point out that even Dr Koop, who worked for the protection of the handicapped newborn in the United States, appears to regard it as plain common sense that there would not be vigorous attempts to save the life of an anencephalic infant. They regard this common sense approach as correct, but as being at odds with the view that all human lives are of equal worth. In another paper, Singer (1985) suggests that merely being human does not confer an intrinsic value to the individual. While normal humans have identifiably 'human' characteristics, such as capacities to reason, to anticipate the distant future, to communicate in a sophisticated way, to be fully self-conscious, these are precisely the characteristics which are lacking in the most severely handicapped. These writers follow their argument to its logical conclusion, i.e. that no newborn infant can in this light be regarded as fully human. They state:

when we kill a newborn infant there is no *person* whose life has begun . . . It is the beginning of the life of the person, rather than of the physical organism, that is crucial so far as the right to life is concerned.

Kuhse and Singer go on to qualify their position by reasoning that there may be a good case for protecting the lives of newborn infants even if, strictly speaking, they do not have a right to life. Since most babies are wanted and loved by their parents, it would constitute a terrible wrong to the baby's parents to kill it. Even if the baby was not wanted by its natural parents and if there was a childless couple eager to adopt and care for the infant, this couple would be wronged by the child being killed. Further, while the infant may not have a right to life, it may have a right to protection from pain, hunger, and cold. Their final conclusion however, is that there is no moral reason why a severely handicapped infant should not be helped to die. I have abbreviated the argument and interested readers are referred to the original articles.

It is an important argument because it represents a trend in thinking which in its full-blown form is intuitively rejected by many, yet which can exert a subtle influence in support of a pragmatic approach to dilemmas affecting human life. The arguments are logical but they operate on false assumptions. The first is, as Singer admits, that the denial of intrinsic value to each individual human being can be argued only from a secular perspective. This, I would argue, has an immediately dehumanizing effect. If God created men and women to reach their fullest humanity in relationship with Him, as Christ's teaching suggests, then to discuss human life and death without reference to God misses a dimension which is at the very heart of humanhood. While for many people spiritual realities may be something of a mystery which they only rarely consider, and while it is true that western society has become increasingly secularized, there is still a tendency, particularly in confronting painful issues, to refer to God, however ill-defined the person's thoughts may be. Further, since Britain is increasingly a multi-racial society, we should bear in mind that in many cultures religion is inextricably linked with the whole of life. There is something fundamental to a sense of meaning in life at stake here.

The second area for disagreement is in the definition of personhood. Assigning particular characteristics to human beings and making these qualifications for personhood is a dangerous practice as it makes us, as human beings and persons, judges of other human beings in a nihilistic sense. It follows that, once we have denied personhood to an individual, we have stripped him or her (or it?) of all rights. Kuhse and Singer seem unusually inconsistent here, in their contention that while newborn infants cannot have a right to continued life, they may have rights to have pain relieved and to be kept warm and fed. 'These rights are not absolute but they indicate what we ought not to do to infants except for overriding reasons.' Since an infant's needs for food, warmth and comfort are needs which he or she seeks to communicate and which are fundamental to his or her bid for the continuance of his or her life, it seems strange to take measures to meet the secondary needs while denying the primary drive for life. A detailed consideration of the organized behaviour of the newborn infant, such as is offered by Schaffer (1977), makes it very hard to accept that such a complex organism, 'programmed' for human interaction, should be denied the title of person. Nurses working with pre-term infants have an intuitive appreciation of their individual personalities. Since human growth and development is a dynamic and continuous process, it makes little sense to say that the beginning of the life of the person is at some other indefinable point much further along the continuum than conception or birth.

The point can be rightly made by all who argue a case for non-treatment of handicapped neonates, that western society has already sanctioned induced abortion, which simply applies the same rules at an earlier stage of development. The fetus below a defined number of weeks gestation is accorded no right to life and is therefore regarded as a non-person. A difficulty here, for the believer and unbeliever alike, is that in this century, for the first time ever, the church itself seems unsure of where it stands. Cameron and Sims (1986) in their discussion of abortion as a crisis in morals and medicine, observe that there are now conscientious Christians who advocate abortion. This is not the place for debating the abortion issue, but it is not irrelevant to our discussion of the right of life of the handicapped newborn. It is interesting that, apart from those who are committed to the argument of the woman's right to choose, most of those who discuss the case for induced abortion preface their remarks to the effect that they do not like the idea of abortion, but . . . It is my belief that allowing the 'buts', real as they are, to guide practice has resulted in a tragic loss of human potential and has eroded the principle of the sanctity of life in a way that is having, and could yet have, very grave consequences in our society.

The concept of personhood then is crucial to the consideration of how we should treat a human being. If we say that a human organism must demonstrate by intelligence, or by self-consciousness, or by a capacity for human relationships (as has been argued by various modern ethicists) that it is a person, in order to merit nurture and protection, we then have *carte blanche* to deny life-saving measures of any kind to the handicapped newborn. It needs to be said, however, that these criteria could also be applied to mentally handicapped, unconscious, autistic, demented adults and others; the possible scenario puts the Holocaust in the shade. If this seems unnecessarily alarmist, consider the degree to which the 'living will' concept has been accepted in Holland and in parts of the United States. A television report in 1986 revealed that of all deaths that occur in Holland each year, fully one-sixth are attributable to euthanasia (Koop, 1987b). It is not such a big step to take from saying that individuals who wish their lives to be terminated should have their request granted, to saying that those who are incapable of such a decision may have it taken on their behalf.

Perhaps the most common criterion used in the attempt to make humane judgements on the issue of treatment of the handicapped newborn is that of quality of life, both for the individual and for the family involved. In relation to the infant, the question to be asked is, what is in the best interests of the child? Where the total motivation is to do good, not harm, to the baby, how vigorously should technology be applied? Virtually all who support the infant's right to life concede that there are situations in which it is right to remove life support apparatus from an irreversibly dying infant and allow it to die in the arms of loving parents (Garland, 1983). They would also argue, however, that the presence of a mental impairment ought not to be allowed to influence decisions regarding surgery. Lusthaus (1985) views the quality of life perspective as putting a value on someone else's life, so that lives that are seen as not worthwhile are thought to be meaningless and less than fully human. Arguing for the rights of people with mental retardation, Lusthaus is clearly concerned by the evidence that potential quality of life was the most important factor among physicians in making decisions about selective medical treatment of infants with Down's syndrome.

FAMILY CONSIDERATIONS

Consideration of the hardship caused to families through having to care for a severely handicapped child clearly influences the decisions made by paediatricians and the outlook of professional and lay people on this difficult subject. Stinson's account of the harrowing experience of parents during prolonged attempts to save their baby's life calls for consideration of the rights and needs of the whole family, including those of children as yet unborn (Stinson and Stinson, 1983). Garland (1983) argues that parents are expected to bear a considerable burden in the ordinary provision of sustenance and nurture for their offspring. There are points, he contends, at which the basic right to life of an individual child, while not abrogated, may be outweighed by the parental right to avoid severe burden and strain on the family's coping strengths. He is very clear however, that this is a liberty which belongs exclusively to the parents, and when it is not exercised health-care providers should act in single-minded pursuit of the infant's best interests. While this is an appealing argument, it does have weaknesses. First, at the point where decisions have to be made about treatment of a handicapped newborn, the parents are emotionally shocked by the impact of bad news immediately following the high of the birth. Second, prediction is difficult, even with the knowledge base and experience of a neonatologist, and most parents have no option but to accept the information they are given by the expert. Thirdly, one has to consider the additional burden of guilt which parents may later experience if they feel that a decision against treatment was theirs alone. Perhaps allowing a family to choose death for a member they feel unable to support is not acceptable to a caring society, but if that is so, society must accept its responsibility in such situations.

While insisting that the best interests of the infant must come first, it is certainly right to widen the focus of concern to the family and the support that may be needed. Central to this is the need for open communication with the parents, and there is evidence that this is increasingly being practised. Garland (1985) insists that the moral demand for open empathetic communication is always present in every case of infant rescue. Also fundamental is the provision of practical help for parents in this situation, and substitute family care for any infant whose parents feel unable to accept the burden of care. We have already considered the economic aspects of intensive care for the newborn and have to admit that our prosperous western society can afford to care for its most vulnerable members. The question is of will more than of resources. The will however, must extend well beyond the critical neonatal period into life-long support if that is what is required.

NURSING ISSUES

The discussion thus far has centred on issues which principally require medical decision-making, but most thinking people would agree with Ian Kennedy that the difficult decisions surrounding the application of modern technology ought not to be left entirely to the medical profession (Kennedy, 1983). Where do nurses figure in the debate? I think that there are several reasons why nurses ought to be informed and hence be aware of the issues involved.

The most obvious reason is that the nurse has to take action according to the decision the doctor has made, whether that is to give intensive care or to withhold technology and offer simple nurture and loving care. One issue arises here which is particularly pertinent to nurses: if the baby is not expected to live, should it still be fed? This is an issue which has had little attention in the nursing literature. It was alluded to recently by Melia (1988) who referred to a case in New York where an infant with Down's syndrome and duodenal atresia was refused treatment by the parents and feeding was withheld. It took 15 days for the infant to die, which as Melia says, is a long time for nurses to be around a hungry dying baby. The feelings and emotions involved are not easily handled. The morality of sanctioning death by starvation must also be questioned. The unacceptability of passive euthanasia is a poor argument for active euthanasia. It might seem more merciful to kill a baby than to starve him or her to death, but these are not the only available solutions to the problem.

Rothenberg (1986) reviewed the recent medical literature and found some writers taking the view that food and fluids are part of the basic care of a patient, along with warmth and skin care, while others included artificial nutrition and hydration, such as nasogastric or intravenous fluids, with technical interventions such as ventilators or haemodialysis. Taking the latter view, it was argued that food and fluids should be withdrawn when no longer beneficial to the patient. The issue is faced most clearly by Callahan (1983) who wrote,

a denial of nutrition may in the long run become the only effective way to make certain that a large number of biologically tenacious patients actually die.

Rothenberg urges paediatric nurses to study the issues and formulate an ethical position so that they will be prepared to meet the situation when it arises. This advice was also given by Dr Koop when he was asked during a conference how a nurse should deal with the situation of being instructed to withhold feeding. As well as thinking through the situation in advance, Dr Koop suggested identifying one or two like-minded people in the unit, and then when the situation arose, going together to the senior nurse and asking to be relieved of the obligation to carry out these duties. As commented elsewhere (Whyte, 1987), the last point is open to question; if one asks to be relieved of these duties, is one simply leaving the responsibility to someone else? Nursing being as it is, there is also the danger that a nurse making such a request will be judged unable to cope and may suffer professionally as a result of his or her action. In the scenario described by Whitelaw (1986), nurses appear to have an equal say with doctors, and it is to be hoped that, with a team approach to care, nurses will be free to contribute to decision-making without fear of victimization if they appear to be swimming against the tide. Group dynamics, however, are extremely powerful, and one can envisage that even in a unit where open communication is practised, it could be extremely hard for a nurse to stand by his or her convictions while he or she was well aware of the weight of medical opinion and that of senior nursing staff on the opposite side of the debate from his or her own. This is a delicate situation which requires a high level of communication skill from all concerned. It underlines the importance of reading, discussing and thinking through one's position, so that one is able to defend it when the need arises.

Rothenberg suggests that in an era where cost containment has become the all-important factor and where society has little empathy for those who are less than physically or neurologically perfect, the nurse may be the most crucial advocate for the patient's survival.

This leads in to a further reason why nurses need to develop and express their views on the rescue of neonates. If they respond to the challenge, they are in a position to act as knowledgeable advocates, whether in individual situations or in exercising their responsibilities as citizens. The public is interested in matters of bio-ethics and is to some extent aware of the complexity of the issues faced. There is, however, a marked tendency to hail technological successes with delight and to ignore the more shadowy area of handicapped babies. Thankfully techniques are all the time advancing and the outlook for tiny infants is improving, but treatments and approaches to care must be kept under close scrutiny.

CONCLUSIONS

A balance must be found between applying whatever technology is available, regardless of cost (physical and emotional as well as financial) and appropriateness, and choosing death as the easier option for a handicapped infant. While my argument has on the whole supported the child's right to life, I fully emphathize with the comment of an experienced nurse in Duff and Campbell's unit, who said of one infant, 'We lost him several weeks ago. Isn't it time to quit?' There does come a time to say enough is enough. Futile treatment is not in the child's best interests. The dilemmas are real and the answers are not obvious in many instances. It is possible, however, to determine principles of treatment, and this was done in 1983 by a group of organizations in America, representing disability and medical interests (Shearer 1984). Within that statement were the following principles:

Throughout their lives, all disabled individuals have the same rights as other citizens, including access to such major societal activities as health care, education and employment.

These rights for all disabled persons must be recognised at birth.

Parents should be given information on available resources to assist in the care of their disabled infant. Society should be informed about the value and worth of disabled persons. Professional organizations, advocacy groups, the government and individual care givers should educate and inform the general public on the care, need, value and worth of disabled infants.

When medical care is clearly beneficial, it should always be provided . . . Considerations such as anticipated and actual limited potential of an individual and present or future lack of community resources are irrelevant and must not determine the decisions concerning medical care . . .

It is ethically and legally justified to withhold medical or surgical procedures which are clearly futile and will only prolong the act of dying. However, supportive care should be provided, including sustenance as medically indicated and relief of pain and suffering. The needs of the dying person should be respected. The family also should be supported in its grieving.

In cases where it is uncertain whether medical treatment will be beneficial, a person's disability must not be the basis for a decision to withhold treatment. At all times during the process when decisions are being made about the benefit or futility of medical treatment, the person should be cared for in the medically most appropriate ways. When doubt exists at any time about whether to treat, a presumption always should be in favour of treatment.

(Association for Retarded Citizens, Washington DC. 1983)

The UKCC Code of Professional Conduct (1984) gives priority to the safeguarding of the interests of individual patients. It is hard ever to be certain that death would be in the interests of another person, except perhaps where that person is already in the process of dying. In that case, the achievement of a 'good death' is within the professional commitment of both doctors and nurses. The argument against a 'quality of life' judgement was poignantly expressed on radio recently by this comment written by foot by a handicapped person in response to a non-handicapped questioner:

I'm me; I only know what it's like to be me; I don't know what it's like to be you, so how can you know what it's like to be me?

I have attempted in this chapter to air a range of views on the subject of infant euthanasia in the context of neonatal intensive care. We all arrive at decisions on ethical dilemmas according to our own beliefs and values, and my own view has doubtless become apparent. It is my hope that, far from stifling debate, this approach will help nurses to think through their own position. In neonatal nursing we deal with patients at the edge of viability and difficult decisions appear in sharp relief. Wisdom, strength, compassion and empathy are needed if nurses are to care sensitively for such vulnerable patients and their families, and take their place responsibly in the caring team.

REFERENCES

Association for Retarded Citizens (1983) Washington, DC.

Budetti, P., McManus, P., Barrano, N. and Heinen, L.A. (1981) Case study 10: The costs and effectiveness of neonatal intensive care. Washington DC, US Government Printing Office. In Garland, M.J. (1983) Rescue unless . . .. A review of the ethics of infant euthanasia *Adv. in Dev. and Behav. Pediatr.*, **4**, 181–203.

Callahan, D. (1983) On feeding the dying. In Rothenberg, L.S. (1986) To feed or not to feed: that is the question and the ethical dilemma. *J. Pediatr. Nurs.*, **1**, 226–9.

Cameron, N.M. de S. and Sims, P.F. (1986) *Abortion: the crisis in morals and medicine.* Inter-Varsity Press, Leicester, England, p 23.

Colen, B.D. and Kerr, K. (1984) Hard Choices: Facing the ethical, legal and financial dilemmas raised by modern medical technology. Reprinted from *Newsday*, April, 15–19.

Duff, R. and Campbell, A.G.M. (1973) Moral and ethical dilemmas in the special-care nursery. *New Eng. J. Med.*, **289**, (25) 890–4.

Garland, M.J. (1983) Rescue, unless . . . a review of the ethics of infant euthanasia. *Adv. in Dev. and Behav. Pediatr.*, **4**, 181–203.

Kennedy, I. (1983) *Unmasking Medicine*. Granada, p 101.

Koop, C.E. (1987a) Life and death and the handicapped newborn. *Ethics and Medicine*, **33**, Rutherford House, Edinburgh, pp 39–44.

Koop, C.E. (1987b) *To Live or Die? Facing decisions at the end of life.* Word (UK) Ltd, Milton Keynes, England, p 7.

Kuhse, H. and Singer, P. (1985) Handicapped babies: a right to life? *Nursing Mirror*, **160**, 8, 17–20.

Lorber, J. (1974) Selective treatment of myelomeningocele: to treat or not to treat. *Pediatr.*, **53**, 307. Cited in Martin, D., (1985, Summer), Withholding treatment from severely handicapped newborns: ethical-legal issues. *Nurs. Admin. Quarterly*, pp 47–56.

Lusthaus, E.W. (1985) Involuntary euthanasia and current attempts to define persons with mental retardation as less than human. *Mental Retardation*, **23**, 3, 148–54.

McIntosh, I. (1987) Inaugural lecture as Professor of Child Life and Health, Edinburgh University.

Melia, K. (1988) An easy death? Everyday ethics. *Nursing Times*, **84**, (8) pp 46–8.

Pomerance, J.J., Urkainski, C.T., Ukra, T., Henderson, D.H., Nash, A.H. and Meredith, J.L. (1978) Cost of living for infants weighing 1000 g or less at birth. *Pediatr.*, **61**, (6) 908–10. In Garland, M.J. (1983) op. cit.

Rosenbloom, L. and Cudmore, R.E. (1985) Spina bifida: do we have the right policies? *Arch. Dis. Childn.*, **60**, 403–4.

Rothenberg, L.S. (1986). To feed or not to feed: that is the question and the ethical dilemma. *J. Pediatr. Nurs.*, **1.4**, 226–9.

Rumbold, G. (1986) *Ethics in Nursing Practice*. Baillière Tindall, Eastbourne, England, p 25.

Schaffer, R. (1977) *Mothering*. Fontana, London.

Shannon, D.C., Crone, R.K., Todres, I.D. and Moorthy, K.S. (1981) Survival, cost of hospitalization, and prognosis in infants critically ill with respiratory distress syndrome requiring mechanical ventilation. Critical Care Medicine. In Garland, M.F. (1983) op. cit.

Shearer, A. (1984) *Everybody's Ethics: what future for handicapped babies?* Campaign for Mentally Handicapped People, London.

Singer, P. (1985) Can we avoid assigning greater value to some human lives than to others? In Laura, R.S. and Ashman, A.F. (eds) *Moral Issues in Mental Retardation*. Croom Helm, London, pp 91–100.

Stinson, R. and Stinson, P. (1983) The long dying of Baby Andrew. In Kuhse, H. and Singer, P. (1985) op. cit.

Whitelaw, A. (1986) Death as an option in neonatal intensive care. *Lancet*

(Aug 9) 328–31.

Whyte, D.A. (1987) Ethics and nursing – Student Forum. *Ethics and Medicine*, **3.3**, Rutherford House, Edinburgh.

UKCC Code of Professional Conduct for the Nurse, Midwife and Health Visitor, 2nd ed (1984) London.

3

Ethical issues in paediatric intensive care nursing

BELINDA ATKINSON

This chapter considers some of the ethical issues associated with care of the small child in the intensive care unit. The discussion of the theory of ethics and underlying values has been left to other writers and the chapter concentrates on the practical problems which may face nurses and staff of other disciplines when caring for such patients. The ethics surrounding the care of a child often involve complex, multi-faceted and emotive issues. The complexity of these issues has increased as technological advances have been made and paediatric patients have been found to respond well to intensive therapy.

Let us begin with some basic statements. Melia (1987) states:

Nurses and doctors have long taken the view that they know best how to treat and care for patients. Indeed, by the nature of the work they do, doctors and nurses have a duty to care for their patients. At the heart of this duty to care is the premise that health professionals should 'do good, and do no harm'.

The International Council for Nurses' (ICN's) *Code for Nurses* states:

the fundamental responsibility of the nurse is fourfold: to promote health; to prevent illness; to restore health and to alleviate suffering.

In the Hippocratic Oath, a doctor promises that the treatments adopted

shall be for the benefit of the patient according to my ability and judgement and not for their hurt or for any wrong.

Maybe this all seems very obvious – in which case why do we need to consider the ethical implications of paediatric intensive care?

Because ethics are important – we all have different beliefs and values – we place differing emphasis on different emotive issues. Ethics are what concern us – we question our practice, why and how we do things and what we are going to achieve by doing so. Ethics mean many different things – there are professional ethics, i.e. how we behave in our work environment; there are ethical committees, such as those concerned with research; and then there are the ethical issues surrounding the care of our patients.

It is not the intention of this chapter to lay down hard and fast rules regarding ethical issues concerning critically ill children; this would not be appropriate, nor would it recognize the individual needs of the child and family. Rather, it is concerned with some of the points which could, and should, be taken into consideration, when faced with the ethical dilemmas surrounding these patients. It can undoubtedly be argued that many of the points raised can also be applied to the adult patient in the intensive care unit, but experience has shown that ethical decisions surrounding children are compounded by the fact that a young patient is involved, because the emotive overtones are always heightened.

It would be appropriate at this stage to consider, albeit briefly, the intensive care unit and the type of patients who may be found there.

Intensive care units have developed rapidly in recent years. Anaesthetic techniques, specialities such as cardiac surgery and neurosurgery, and respiratory therapy have all increased in their scope and complexity, and with them have come advances in technology and new practices. These developments, plus the rapid therapeutic advances seen today, have meant that extremely sick patients can be cared for; patients who would probably have had little or no chance of surviving only a few years ago (Atkinson, 1987a). This has inevitably led to problems of its own.

The rationale behind concentrating critically ill patients in one area is that this will also concentrate specialist resources and equipment – with the aim of providing the best possible care for the very sick patient. Initially these resources tended to be concentrated in a single general intensive care unit, as suggested by Tinker (1978) – there are many similarities in the care of various disorders; irrespective of the nature of the primary illness, all could be managed in a single general intensive therapy unit.

Advances in many specialities have led to the setting up of specialist units. These may have problems in that they are expensive to run, and they dilute the experienced staffing resources available (McLachlan, 1984), but they may be more geared to the needs of specific groups of critically ill patients – and this is undoubtedly so in the case of the critically ill child. The need for this type of provision for children has recently been the subject of a report from the British Paediatric Association (B.P.A., 1986). Davies (1987) and Coles (1987) describe the 'ideal' environment and the basic principles of care which should be aimed for when caring for sick children in intensive care units, and their families.

Children who require admission to intensive care units are generally extremely ill, often with complex diseases. In many cases, the child's condition may have worsened suddenly, precipitating admission to the unit (Hazinski, 1987a). Many children will be ventilator dependent, unable to communicate, and attached to a whole myriad of supportive equipment and therapy. Most of the procedures performed on children in intensive care units are unfamiliar to the child, and many are uncomfortable and sometimes painful.

The conditions necessitating admission to the intensive care unit vary considerably, but can be very generally grouped as follows:

Major surgery, e.g. cardiothoracic surgery or neurosurgery;
Trauma;
Non-accidental injury;
Near drowning;
Neurological conditions, e.g. Reye's syndrome;
Upper respiratory tract obstructure or infection;
Cardio–respiratory arrest;
Infectious diseases;
Repiratory problems, e.g. asthma.

This list is by no means comprehensive, and there are other conditions which, from time to time, may necessitate the admission of a child to the intensive care unit. In addition, local hospital policy may vary as to whether children with certain conditions are admitted to the intensive care unit or cared for in the paediatric wards, or a high dependency area. This chapter, however, is concerned with the most critically ill children in this range.

What makes intensive care units different from other nursing units? Many would argue that they are not, and that today many different areas of patient care can be considered to be specialities.

However, there are differences between intensive care units and general ward areas, in the following respects:

1. The higher turnover of patients and the not infrequent deaths;
2. The problems of communicating directly with many of the patients;
3. The perceived moral and ethical dilemmas regarding treatment, often highlighted in such units;
4. The higher ratio of nurses to patients;
5. The high level of contact and involvement of the nurse with the family;
6. The wide range of patient's ages and conditions which the nurse is expected to be able to care for;
7. The cost of care – it has been estimated that it costs four to five times more to keep a patient in an intensive care unit per day, than in a general ward.

    Intensive care has to be considered not only for its cost in its own right, but also in terms of the proportion of total financial resources allocated to an individual hospital which the unit uses;
8. The inherent hostility and unfriendliness of the environment.

Perhaps one of the most significant characteristics of an intensive care unit, with specific reference to paediatrics and ethical issues, is summarized by Stinson *et al* (1979) as follows:

The complexity of modern newborn intensive care (and other forms of intensive care) demands the participation and teamwork of a large group of individual personalities with different degrees of knowledge, competence, experience, sensitivity and judgement. They will have different views on purely technical matters quite apart from widely varying opinions on ethics and law.

With the kind of mix described, it is important that there is a clearly defined leader and a strong sense of team spirit. This will be relevant to ethical decision-making, but it has also been supported by the findings, of a study by Knaus *et al* (1982). Amongst other findings they discovered that there was a tendency towards favourable patient outcome statistics for those units that had clearly defined leaders with well defined responsibilities, an interest in the training and development of their staff, and specific policies and guidelines for the admission, treatment and care of patients.

Before examining specific problems, it is worth dwelling briefly on the criteria for admission to intensive care units, because these may have significant relevance to later problems.

It is not general practice in the UK to operate cut-off limits for admissions to intensive care units. McLachlan (1984) states that an admission policy is deemed necessary to make sensible use of an expensive resource and that it is also conducive to good management practice. In reality, most admission policies in operation seem to be concerned more with the actual mechanics of admission, rather than with the conditions involved. Some general guidelines have been suggested by several leading authorities, amongst them Tinker (1978):

1. The physiological disturbance should be judged to be reversible;
2. There may be a problem where acute-on-chronic illness is concerned, and the possible outcome of treatment must be considered in depth;
3. Patients should not be admitted solely for 'heavy' nursing.

Melia (1980) suggests that in some cases, where life supporting treatment has been initiated –

once the great save is over, the implications of the life saving actions slowly become apparent. Heroic deeds are always more easily performed than reversed.

We are urged to remember two points:

1. Life of any quality is not necessarily better than no life at all;
2. Decisions about life saving are often dictated by medical possibilities and are made in the unsuitable surroundings of modern hospital technology (Melia, 1980).

Let us now discuss some specific issues arising from the care of the child in the intensive care unit.

The first question that needs to be addressed is – who is best qualified to represent the interests of the child and to be the child's advocate? A review of the literature demonstrates that this question has been widely examined, with no one conclusive answer. However, I would like to examine the problem from three view-points, with brief mention of a fourth for completeness:

1. The parents;
2. The medical staff;
3. The nursing staff;
4. Other interested parties.

Generally, it would be considered that the parents have ownership of the child – and therefore, undoubtedly, the most right to represent their child's interests. They have to carry the personal consequences of any decision, and the long-term implications of treatment will, in almost every case, have the maximum impact on them. However, there may be occasions when, because of the intimate relationship between parents and child, they find it difficult to be involved in such decisions, and we must always have respect for their mental state and their consequent ability to be involved in such crucial decisions. Perhaps it is these latter considerations which have given rise to some of the debate and concern surrounding this issue.

Erickson *et al* (1987) state:

In infancy and early childhood the rights of parents and their ability to act in the child's best interests ideally exist in a delicate balance. In this age group, decision-making by proxy is well accepted. Although the legal right of the parent or guardian to make decisions in the presumed best interest of the child is undisputed, neither blood ties nor legal guardianship ensures that the best interests of the child are always foremost or that objective decisions will be made.

The authors continue their debate to suggest that the practitioner must act as an advocate for the child, but refrain from projecting personal values or beliefs onto the parental decision-maker. We will discuss information further at a later stage, but it is also suggested by these writers that, in the case of older children, the legal rights of the parent must be weighed against the autonomous rights of the maturing individual. This implies that, where possible, gaining the child's agreement when a decision or plan is being made is desirable, this is referred to by some as 'informed assent'. This means that the parents retain ultimate responsibility for decision-making, but the child is not excluded from the process.

Literature from the USA suggests that 'although parents are usually viewed as being the most capable of making decisions for their infants, a debate exists regarding whether parents, professionals, or the courts should have the final say about health care and life-and-death issues relating to the 0–2 years age group' (Verzemnieks and Nash, 1984).

Writing from the parental point of view, Stinson and Stinson (1983) stated:

We feel that we, as the child's parents, were more likely to have feelings of concern for (his) suffering than the necessarily detached medical staff, busy with scores of other cases and 'interesting' projects – who can determine whether, or at what point, the child's true advocate is the person proclaiming his right to life or the person proclaiming his right to death?

Later in the same article, these authors express a fear of

the prospect of having to care for the rest of our lives for a pathetically handicapped, retarded child.

Indeed, many decisions will have the most significant long-term effects upon the parents; and decisions must never be made unilaterally by those who do not have to live with the consequences.

The involvement of medical practitioners takes a different slant. It is considered natural and necessary that health professionals seek to preserve life. Indeed, the majority of our efforts are directed toward measures, even heroic measures, that will cure illness and delay death (Fowler, 1987). Technology has aided us in this, and we will return to this aspect later. It has been said by some that the situation now exists in which it is very easy to turn on a respirator – and almost impossible to turn one off (Stinson and Stinson, 1983).

In the same vein, Cassem, writing in 1980, stated

stopping treatment is ethically no different than starting it . . . Ethically, treatments that will reverse illness and restore health are regarded as necessary. The treatments that cannot reverse illness in a moribund patient are not necessary, and if the benefit versus suffering indicates that more suffering will result from application of treatment, it is contra-indicated.

The question that is raised time and time again in such context is 'at what point does one stop?' There is never an easy answer to this. Sometimes it is difficult for the doctor to win – he or she may on the one hand be accused of giving up too easily, or on the other, of prolonging life to such an extent that the resulting degree of disability makes life intolerable for the patient.

Todres wrote in 1985:

Physicians working in intensive care units are faced with an agonizing dilemma . . . Medical training has taught and prepared the physician to preserve life, and to relieve pain and suffering. In the intensive care unit, these aims are sometimes contradictory but at all times the physician should consider the best interests of the child.

The physician must ensure that the medical aspects of the case in question – diagnosis, treatment and prognosis – are as fully informed as possible, so that the facts can be clarified and communicated to those who need to know. Undoubtedly, uncertainty exists in many areas of medical knowledge, and the physician must aim to limit these areas of uncertainty to the best of his or her ability. Only then can he or she have any claim to act as the child's advocate in the decision-making process.

There are occasions when it may be appropriate to continue therapy if there is doubt concerning the outcome or effect of such therapy, until further evaluation can assist those involved to reach a decision.

It is also important that nurses continue to act as advocates for children, because decision-making must involve all the members of the health-care team as well as the parents; this must include the nursing staff involved in the care of the child. For paediatric nurses, concern over ethical issues and their correct resolution is not a professional luxury, but an integral part of their work (Brykczyńska, 1985). Experienced nurses often have a valuable contribution to make in the decision-making process – many have previous experience of similar cases and, having constant access to the child and its parents, observation of the coping mechanisms of the parents, and their thought processes, is generally possible. This supports the need for a good rapport to be developed between the family and nursing staff, so that these aspects of behaviour can be noted.

Nurses in intensive care units who are involved in such crucial decisions must take responsibility, rather than go along with the general trend, if they believe a decision is unethical (Verzemnieks and Nash, 1984). Only by being properly prepared will they be able to do this, and nurses must learn not to shy away from ethical issues. The introduction of ethical concepts at an early stage in training is paramount, and this should be followed through at all stages of the career. Formal societies, journal clubs, ethical rounds, study days and discussion groups may all assist in this; but in reality it is likely that the ethical issues surrounding the definition of death, withholding and/or terminating treatment, organ donation, suffering and dignity – as well as the allocation of resources, will continue to combine to present profound ethical problems for nurses caring for critically ill children. It is therefore necessary that nurses develop the ability to reason objectively.

Finally, in some societies, there may be other interested parties involved in ethical decision-making. Lack of direct experience on the part of the author does not permit a detailed discussion of this aspect – but parties that come to mind are those involved in transplant surgery, and/or legal personnel in cases such as insurance claims, unusual circumstances etc. These individuals do not generally have direct ownership of the child, and therefore it can be argued that they are not best qualified to represent the child, but they may indeed have a contribution to make, or a profound effect upon the decision-making process.

With regard to the personnel involved in ethical decision-making, Doudera and Peters (1982) summarize the need for an inter-disciplinary approach to all ethical decisions in the clinical area, by suggesting that 'after all, life and death decisions are not just for doctors and nurses. Indeed, they are for everyone.'

There are one or two other aspects concerning decision-making in the paediatric intensive care unit, which are worthy of consideration.

Problems can occur when there are conflicting beliefs between the parties involved. This may be, for example, between nursing and medical staff; or medical staff and the parents. Two main points should be considered: first, decisions must be made by those who are actively involved in the care of the child. Todres (1985) reminds us that 'arm-chair decision makers may be part of the problem, rather than a solution to the problem'.

Problems can arise in the intensive care unit when, for example, the referring team wish to be involved in decision-making concerning their patient, but do not play an active part in the child's care, and perhaps visit the unit infrequently, if at all. It is probably sensible if some reference to authority for decision-making is included as part of the admission policy to the unit, and the lines of responsibility for the management of the child are clearly defined, taking into account the fact that others may want and need to contribute to any significant decisions. There is no place for ivory-tower decision-making in the intensive care unit; decisions are for real, and must be made in that light.

Secondly, if there are conflicting beliefs – discussions and explanations are urgently required so that it can be ascertained and understood why the difference in opinion exists and the approach to the problem can, if necessary be modified.

Probably the hardest conflicts to cope with are those between the parents and the medical or nursing staff. An example comes to mind from some years ago, where a child had complex cardiac surgery for a congenital defect. This type of surgery was very much in its infancy then; the case became very complicated in the post-operative period, and there was much conflict between the various medical staff involved who wished to continue treatment, in the firm belief that this was the right thing to do and was what the parents wanted.

In fact, this was not the case, and the parents had sensed very early on that their young child was not going to survive. Eventually, a member of the nursing staff from the ward where the parents were resident approached the intensive care unit staff, and reported that the parents were beseeching her to ask the medical staff to discontinue treatment. They did not wish to prolong their child's end, and believed that the best course of action for the child was to discontinue treatment. The appropriate dialogue between those involved then started, but obviously too late. In this case nature intervened, as is so often the case – and the child died relatively peacefully within 24 hours.

The case involved, of which I have given only the briefest of sketches, illustrated gross communication problems, and a significant conflict of opinions as to what was best for the child.

It is always easy to be wise after the event, and one would hope that with increased openness with families, and awareness of the need for good communications all round, that this type of problem would be a rare occurrence now. Even though these decisions are difficult, we may have to accept on occasions that the parents may not actually want treatment. Encouraging multiple participation in decision-making is essentially healthy, but may lead in turn to a difficulty of its own – that of arriving at one decision.

This also leads us to another problem with particular relevance to the paediatric intensive care unit – that of the constraints of time. When dealing with a child in the intensive care setting who is acutely ill, complex decisions often need to be made in a very short space of time. Care always has to be taken that all the relevant facts are examined, despite this additional external constraint.

Time does not only put pressure on the parents; Ashworth (1976) reminds us that the intensive therapy nurse is constantly aware that if she is even a few minutes late in noticing and interpreting correctly changes in the information signals which bombard her from the patient and the numerous bits of surrounding equipment, then this may affect the patient's well-being or even life.

Closely linked with this, in respect of decision-making, is objectivity, Verzemnieks *et al* (1984) refer to the fact that

parental stress at the time the diagnosis is made influences ability to make decisions.

We are reminded that provision of adequate information and time for parents to synthesize and deal with their anger and guilt is essential; and yet we have seen how difficult this may be in a life-threatening situation.

Decisions may be further complicated in that selectively deciding to withdraw a particular aspect of treatment may not automatically put an end to suffering, and further confusion and guilt feelings may occur when this suffering continues.

We must always consider the ability of the parents, in terms of their mental state and objectivity, to be involved in such crucial decisions. We need to listen and support, and as nurses we have to remember that the state of the parents may well place an added strain on relationships between them and members of the health-care team at such times.

At this stage, mention should be made of those parents who are playing dual roles, i.e. they may be a parent, and, by profession, a member of a health-care team. There are two dangers here; first, the objectivity of the parents may be influenced by prior knowledge, and they may well have particular difficulty participating in decisions. Secondly, there is always a risk that insufficient information may be given – as it is assumed they 'already know'. It is vital to assess what their knowledge base is, with reference to the particular condition in question.

First and foremost, the individual is the parent of a critically ill child, and should therefore be treated and supported as such.

We should now turn to some other aspects of paediatric intensive care, which tend to pose problems giving rise to concern. Some will encompass issues on which we have already touched, and may be used to broaden the scope of the individual issue.

It is, for example, necessary to consider the impact of modern technological developments with regard to ethical issues. There are perhaps two main aspects involved; first, technological advances have meant that we can now treat conditions of childhood, which were previously considered not treatable. Congenital neurological and cardiac conditions are undoubtedly fine examples, but this is also true of other congenital abnormalities and serious childhood illnesses. As previously alluded to it is now relatively easy to support life, but we need always to bear in mind the possible quality of life that may result from such treatment, and the long-term implications for the child, parents, health-care resources and society generally.

Technology has also worked for us though, in respect of ethical decisions, because in many cases we are now able to make better informed diagnoses, and assess medical conditions more accurately. This means that there should in many instances be a clearer idea regarding prognosis, and therefore whether treatment is possible and/or appropriate. One example of this is the diagnosis of cerebral death.

Cerebral death is a particularly difficult concept in childhood. In adult medicine, there are now well accepted guidelines for the diagnosis of cerebral death (DHSS, 1983; Pallis, 1982). However, it is generally considered that the brain of a young child has more resilience, and therefore may recover despite evidence of extensive neurological injury (Verzemnieks and Nash, 1984). There are documented instances of children recovering from significant neurological insults, and this has led to problems in itself, i.e. it can be very difficult to be involved in decisions to discontinue treatment, if there is this faint glimmer of hope; but on the other hand it is equally difficult to balance this with reality and prolong the life of a child through artificial means, if the general clinical picture holds little hope for recovery.

The criteria for brain stem death vary slightly from country to country. The Code of Practice – Cadaveric Organs for Transplantation (1983) – outlines those used in the UK at present. The tests used to diagnose cerebral death are summarized as follows, certain preconditions having been met:

1. No pupillary response to light;
2. Absent corneal reflex;
3. Absent vestibulo-ocular reflexes;
4. No response to painful stimuli;

5. No gag reflex;
6. No respiratory movements.

(Keogh, 1987)

These tests are performed by two practitioners, and repeated twice. Neither practitioner should be a member of a team involved with organ transplantation, if this is contemplated. Generally, the time of death is recorded as the time that the second definitive set of brain stem tests occur – not following the retrieval procedure of organs for transplantation.

Nursing the child who is thought to be, or has been actively diagnosed to be brain dead, is one of the most stressful aspects of paediatric intensive care nursing. Not only must the nurse support the family, but he or she must also cope objectively with his or her own feelings and emotions. The nurse must always remember that, even when a decision has been made to donate organs, his or her prime responsibility lie with the child and family in his or her care.

This leads us on to discuss the paediatric donor; and, indeed, no discussion of ethical issues in paediatric intensive care would be complete without this. As transplantation techniques have become increasingly sophisticated, so the ethical and moral issues have become the subject of public concern. Media interest and coverage have heightened such discussions. We will concentrate on some of the general issues involved.

First, there is again a problem in that a child is involved. Secondly, that particular child may be a highly desirable donor because of height, weight and blood group matching – the first two being more relevant for paediatric recipients. At the time of writing there is a national shortage of paediatric donors and this may at times put pressure onto an already difficult situation.

The health-care team in the intensive care unit should discuss organ donation openly with the families of children who are declared brain dead, and who are considered suitable for organ donation. Hazinski (1987b) states categorically that

family members should never feel pressured to agree to organ donation – the health-care team should merely ensure that the family's refusal is an informed one.

It may be helpful to involve the local transplant co-ordinator in the discussions, because he or she will be in the position to answer many of the questions that the parents may wish to ask. Issues such as whether the child's body will be disfigured, and whether the procedure will delay the funeral arrangements are often uppermost, and need to be answered honestly and in an informed manner. Adequate explanation of the issues involved, and support of the family at this time, requires commitment to the philosophy of transplantation and organ donation by all members of the health-care team who are involved in the process.

The third issue involved is the problem of exactly when to approach the parents. Many children who are admitted to the intensive care unit and become potential organ donors, have been admitted urgently as the result of, for example, a road traffic accident. The relationship between health-care professionals and parents may not have had time to build up to the desired level – and often it is the nurses at the bedside who will gain the first insight into how a particular family views the concept of organ donation.

The opinion of many is that the right time to approach the parents is between the two sets of cerebral death tests, so that the reasons for doing the tests are not misconstrued. The concept of cerebral death itself needs exploring with the family in early discussions of the child's prognosis, and a clearcut definition needs to be provided. Consistency in approach and terminology is vital, between all involved in the child's care.

Obviously, it is necessary to adapt differing approaches to different situations. It may be that the parents make the approach themselves – some feel comforted in their loss by knowing that they can help another child. If an approach is made by the parents in this way, it is up to all concerned to ensure that the organs are used – we may be perceived as failing the parents in their wishes if we do not.

This is important for nurses as well, as the nurse will have had to help the family cope with the child's sudden and severe injury, support the family through the diagnosis and death, and provide skilled support to maintain organ perfusion in the case of organ donation.

Following all of this skilled and devoted care, the nurse can not look forward to the recovery of the patient, but must be able to derive satisfaction from knowing that the donor family was supported through a terrible experience. In addition, the nurse will know that a potentially life-saving organ was provided for another child.

(Hazinski, 1987b).

Media publicity has advantages and disadvantages. It is suggested that the number of paediatric organ donors has increased following some fairly notable media attention. This has to be seen as positive and good for those children for whom transplantation is the only hope of leading a normal life. However, excessive publicity has made relatives of some potential donors reticent, and we always need to ensure their understanding of the situation – often difficult in such circumstances.

Lastly, there are, as always, the emotional overtones. Transplantation is not yet universally accepted as the right thing by everyone. Resources are still relatively scarce, so that only a few patients will have the chance of receiving an organ transplant. The statistics are generally improving, at least for adults – and in this case it may well be argued that the economic advantages in the long-term are worth it if the individual can maintain a normal lifestyle and play a full part in society. However, the situation appears to be a little different in paediatrics – there are far-reaching issues, the implications of which have yet to become fully apparent.

At present, there is widespread debate about such issues as 'opting out' or 'required request'. Whilst these may be seen to be the right thing to do by many, it can also be argued that there is no substitute for enhanced education and awareness, not only of the general public, but also of the medical and nursing professions. The well-being of the patients in our care is our first priority and, indeed, we have an obligation to assist the dying individual toward a peaceful death (Henderson, 1966). At times there is nothing more that can be done for a particular child and in these cases perhaps we should consider that

transplantation is now a routine form of treatment and by working together we can benefit all our patients.

(Keogh, 1987).

There are other groups of patients in the paediatric intensive care unit who may precipitate ethical dilemmas for their carers. One such group are children who are admitted to such units following obvious or suspected non-accidental injury.

The main problems for the nurse are first that the child may have appalling or unusual injuries, and secondly that there may be very difficult family circumstances to cope with. Nurses have to remember that they are primarily there to care, and not to judge.

However, these cases may produce problems of their own, in that a contradiction of some of the principles discussed earlier may result.

For instance, we have seen how parents are given the right to act in their child's best interests in most situations. In cases such as non-accidental injury, parental authority may not be absolute – this may be evidenced by court or other decisions reversing parental authority to make treatment decisions, as well as by child abuse/neglect laws (Verzemnieks and Nash, 1984).

Contained within most moral codes and certainly within those of the major world religions, is the idea that to take human life, at least in most circumstances, is wrong (Rumbold, 1986). In fact we have seen at the very beginning of this chapter that a major part of the philosophy of health-care is to relieve suffering and restore health. The nurse is therefore caught in a dilemma when dealing with non-accidental injury. On the one hand she has possibly a very sick child to care for and parents fraught with confusion, emotions and difficulties, and on the other she has to balance objectivity, compassion and support against what she as an individual may believe is vehemently wrong – often truely a challenge to her own values and moral beliefs/principles.

We have also to consider what might be referred to as the unpopular patient, who might be a child or its parents. In the case of a child, this term is applied very loosely, and generally refers to the child who is physically affected in a way that makes him or her difficult to cope with on a day-to-day basis. Examples are the child who is infectious, requiring barrier nursing; the child who has open or broken down wounds; or the child who is grossly physically disfigured such as a burned child. In these cases the nurse may have an underlying feeling of difficulty in coping with the care of such children, and may actually feel that he or she does not want to be allocated the care of such a patient. Not only must he or she cope with these feelings and difficulties, but must also present an air of confidence and objectiveness in dealing with the family.

The final group of children who may pose severe ethical dilemmas in the intensive care unit are those who have been determined as hopeless cases. In some respects we have already alluded to such problems, and perhaps we have come full circle, and returned to the problem of whether to treat, and, if so, when to stop.

Fowler (1987) suggests that it is difficult to love a patient to death, and this theme is also explored by Ashworth (1982). She stated that some studies have shown that death of a patient is ranked by nurses as one of the most stressful factors in intensive care nursing. This stress is said to be increased when there are unresolved ethical dilemmas or conflicts over the prolongation of life, and can be reduced by open discussion and decision-making between nurses and doctors, with good communication with patients' visitors.

Much work has been done in the USA concerning the issues involved in the withdrawal of treatment. I quote from this, because although not applicable in UK law, the basic concepts are important.

In 1983 the President's Commission for the Study of Ethical Problems in Medicine report was published, entitled *Deciding to Forego Life-Sustaining Treatment*. This document forms an ethical core for decision-making in practice, and for the development of professional position statements and institutional policies or guidelines (Fowler, 1987). There is, as yet, no similar publication in the UK, although the above report is often cited in the literature.

The Judicial Council of the American Medical Association (1984) states:

The consideration of the physicians should be what is the best for the individual patient and not the avoidance of a burden to the family or society. Quality of life is a factor to be considered in determining what is best for the individual . . . Withholding or removing life support means is ethical provided that the normal care given an individual who is ill, is not discontinued.

Finally, the President's Commission (1983) states:

A justification that is adequate for not commencing a treatment is also sufficient for ceasing it.

Most importantly, all children should receive total, respectful and supportive care, even when no further medical care is desirable or electively chosen. Fowler (1987) tells the story of the death of the Rabbi Judah the Prince. The Prince was dying from a terminal gastrointestinal disease. His female servant, a woman of unquestioned piety and moral character, prayed for his death, while the rabbis surrounding him prayed for life. The prayers of the rabbis were efficacious in prolonging the agonizing dying of the Prince. Distressed by the action of the rabbis, the woman dropped a clay pot from above, shattering it in their midst. Startled from their prayers, the rabbis ceased praying, and the soul of the Prince departed.

Fowler suggests that sometimes, whether from pain, pride, pressure, or a misinterpretation of either ethics or the law, the clay pot must shatter in our midst to jolt us into withdrawing treatment from an irretrievably dying and suffering patient. She concludes by summarizing that in these sorts of situations, we should not be led into treating a patient for whom treatment is futile or undesired – 'treatment should cease before the pot is ever broken'.

Cassem (1980) states that, when illness is judged irreversible – 'life is not the absolute good, nor is death the absolute evil'.

Before we consider how to help intensive care nurses cope with some of the problems that have been discussed, there are two other issues at stake. The first is the responsibility of the nurse, and his or her obligations when caring for critically ill children.

The *UKCC Code of Professional Conduct* gives us the essentials of some broad guidelines:

Each registered nurse, midwife and health visitor is accountable for his or her practice and, in the exercise of professional accountability shall:
1. Act always in such a way as to promote and safeguard the well-being and interests of patients/clients;
2. Ensure that no action or omission on his/her part or within his/her sphere of influence is detrimental to the condition or safety of patients/clients.

Ashworth (1976) suggests that if we take part in life-maintaining procedures, we must also accept some responsibility for the quality of that life and the quality of care given to those who survive. The *ICN Code* (1973) addresses the obligation of the nurse to participate in continual learning to enhance clinical practice and competence.

Intensive therapy is constantly changing – new techniques are being developed and therapeutic boundaries crossed. Entrusted to our care are some of the very sickest, most highly dependent patients in the health-care system, and we therefore have an obligation to maintain the highest and safest standards of care possible for these children and their families. This involves constant learning and updating to increase our knowledge and improve our practice.

Also inherent in paediatric intensive care nursing is the concept of the extended role in the nurse. This type of nursing, coupled with modern technology, has frequently stimulated nurses to undertake more complex tasks, and develop new skills. Many references may be found in the literature relating to the extended role, among them Rowden (1987). Rowden stresses that the extension of the role must be in the interests of patient care, and must not be introduced as a means of providing quick or cheap solutions to manpower problems. Nurses, he states, cannot and must not be expected to undertake any role extension without adequate training.

Ashworth takes an interesting view of the extended role of the nurse. She states categorically that

whenever we take on a new responsibility for ourselves or our staff we must be aware of its implications as well as competent to accept it. Our technical competence has increased rapidly in recent years, and many nurses now cope calmly and competently with situations which many of their seniors would be reluctant to face.

She considers whether, in the midst of all the technological advancement, we have always maintained our 'respect for the beliefs, values and customs of the individual?' The example quoted is whether we would always remember an Orthodox Jew's dietary restriction, even when he is tube fed? She asks whether this matters – and concludes that it does – 'if we believe that our patients have a right to expect that we will respect those things which they (or their parents and families) hold to be important' (Ashworth, 1976). Certainly an interesting viewpoint, worthy of consideration and respect.

My final issue concerns cost. Should cost be a consideration in ethical decision-making? In most countries of the world today, financial considerations have become a concern in intensive care and health-care generally. We have to consider both immediate and long-term costs, and I would suggest that we will see financial considerations, distasteful as they may be to many, brought into ethical decision-making in the future.

In an increasingly cost-conscious climate, the financial implications of intensive care are a major factor. There is no escaping the fact that intensive care units are expensive to run, therefore value for money has to be considered (McLachlan, 1984). Intensive care has to be considered not only for its cost in its own right, but also in terms of the proportion of total financial resources allocated to individual hospitals, which the unit consumes (Atkinson, 1987b).

Tinker (1978) suggests that these high costs lead to questions concerning the ethical implications of concentrating so much of the available resources on a relatively small number of patients but that, despite the fact that the cost of intensive care is well recognized, any restriction will have a profound effect on patient care and survival.

Currently, work is being done on a new measure of quality of life which combines length of survival with an attempt to measure the quality of that survival. This measure is the 'Quality Adjusted Life Year' (Williams, 1985). The advantages and disadvantages of this method are discussed by Harris (1987), and some of the ethical issues involved are referred to in this discussion. Essentially, the decisions involved concern choices regarding an individual's life, condition and age – all therefore could have ethical implications. Williams (1985) states that

it is the responsibility of everyone to discriminate whenever necessary to ensure that our limited resources go where they will do the most good.

It is early days yet, but I suspect that we will hear more of this measure, together with the moral and ethical discussions which are likely to ensue.

Finally, how can we help nurses in paediatric intensive care units to cope with ethical issues, and how can awareness of ethical issues generally be increased? I have used as my framework for suggestions ideas put forward by Brykczyńska (1985), because many of these are relevant to intensive care units.

First, the concept of ethical rounds. This is examined with specific reference to intensive care units by Davis (1979). These rounds give the opportunity for a group of staff to meet, preferably in a room separate from the unit, to discuss individual cases and the ethical issues involved. Leadership of the group may be from any discipline, but should be informed and objective. Most importantly, the discussion at such a meeting should be confidential to those involved, so that all may be free to share their opinions and concerns.

More junior nurses tend now to view it as their right to be assisted in coping with ethical and moral dilemmas in their work. Undoubtedly, as senior nurses, this is our responsibility. However, it should never be forgotten that more senior members of staff also need guidance and support and this has to be provided – indeed some studies (Amis, 1978) have shown that senior nurses in ICU's have experienced more stress than junior nurses, and others (Hingley, 1986) have found that, even at senior nurse level, death and dying still caused a considerable degree of stress.

Secondly, ward teaching sessions can be planned to include discussion of ethical issues. These can be led by experienced nurses, and possibly planned in conjunction with the school of nursing. In addition, attendance at conferences or seminars where ethical issues are to be discussed should be encouraged. Brykczyńska suggests that perhaps groups of hospitals could combine together to organize such events. Alternatively, input from professional nursing bodies would be desirable – especially from the specialist nursing bodies concerned with paediatrics and intensive care – the Royal College of Nursing Forums, the British Association of Critical Care Nurses, and the Neonatal Nurses Group amongst others.

Thirdly, nursing libraries and/or individual units could help to promote awareness of ethical issues by subscribing to any relevant journals and purchasing books concerned with nursing ethics. The formation of journal clubs may also assist.

Good team collaboration within the intensive care unit is also important, and has been referred to already. A sensitivity between colleagues may help to identify when team members are having difficulty coping with a particular problem. This need is not only specific to nursing, but to all disciplines involved in intensive care.

At the fourth World Congress of Intensive Care Medicine, held in Israel in 1985, it was apparent that there was a marked increase in discussion of such matters as cost and ethical issues. Perhaps technology has now left us at a point where these issues are paramount, and we need to look very closely at guidelines for the ethical practice of intensive care.

The ethical issues concerning children are compounded by the age of the patient involved, but they will not go away, and silence will not make them any easier to cope with. There are no absolute solutions, and there is very rarely a finite answer as to what is reasonable. Only by exposing the issues and discussing them, and by educating our staff, will we prepare them to cope with the ethical dilemmas of modern paediatric intensive care.

REFERENCES

Amis, M. Cited by Cowper-Smith (1978) Intensive care needed for all in ITU's. *Nursing Times*, **74**, 1158.

Ashworth, P. (1976) Ethics in the ITU. *Nursing Times*, Nov, 153–6.

Ashworth, P. (1982) Intensive care – when intensive care fails. *Nursing*, 1st Series, **34**, 1481-2.

Atkinson, B.L. (1987a) The intensive care unit. *Nursing*, 3rd Series, **15**, 547-51.

Atkinson, B.L. (1987b) Management of the intensive care unit. *Nursing*, 3rd Series, **16**, 583-9.

British Paediatric Association (1986) Chairman: D.J. Matthew *Report of a Working Party on Paediatric Intensive Care*. British Paediatric Association, London.

Brykczyńska, G.M. (1985) Ethical issues in paediatric nursing. *Nursing*, 2nd Series **40**, 1184-6.

Cassem, N.H. (1980) Psychiatrie. In E. Rubenstein and D.D. Federman (eds) Section 13. *Scientific American Medicine*, New York.

Coles, J.M. (1987) The child in the intensive care unit. *Nursing*, 3rd Series **16**, 608-11.

Davies, C.J. (1987) He's not my baby any more. *Nursing*, 3rd Series **13**, 498-502.

Davis, A.J. (1979) Ethics rounds with intensive care nurses. *Nursing Clinics of North America*, **14** (1), 45-55.

DHSS (1983), *Cadaveric Organs for Transplantation; A Code of Practice including the diagnosis of brain stem death*. DHSS, London.

Doudera, A.E. and Peters, J.D. (1982) *Legal and Ethical Aspects of Treating Critically and Terminally Ill Patients*. AUPH Press, Ann Arbor, Michigan.

Erickson, S. and Hopkins, M.A. (1987) Gray areas: informed consent in paediatric and comatose adult patients. *Heart and Lung*, **16** (3), 323-5.

Fowler, M.D. (1987) And the Rabbi Judah the Prince died: on the withdrawal of treatment. *Heart and Lung*, **16** (5), 576-8.

Harris, J. (1987) QALYfying the value of life. *J. Med. Ethics*, **13**, 117-123.

Hazinski, M.F. (1987a) Methods of improving critical care expertise of the general pediatric nurse. *Pediatric Nursing*, **13** (4), 260.

Hazinski, M.F. (1987b) Pediatric organ donation: responsibilities of the critical care nurse. *Pediatric Nursing*, **13** (5), 354-7.

Henderson, V. (1966) *The Nature of Nursing: A definition and its implications for practice, research and education*. The Macmillan Company, New York.

Hingley, P. (1986) Burnout at senior level. *Nursing Times*, **82** (31), 28-9.

ICN, (1973) *Code for Nurses: Ethical Concepts applied to Nursing*. International Council of Nurses, Geneva.

Judicial Council, American Medical Association (1984) *Current opinions of the Judicial Council of the American Medical Association*, The Association, Chicago.

Keogh, A. (1987) Transplantation and organ donation. *Nursing*, 3rd series **16**, 590–2.

Knaus, W.A., Draper, E.A. and Wagner, P.D. (1982) Evaluating outcome from intensive care: a preliminary multihospital comparison. *Critical Care Medicine* **10**, 491.

Liddell, G. (1982) Death of a child. *Nursing*, 1st Series **34**, 1496–7.

McLachlan, G. (1984) The intensiveness of care. *Nursing Mirror*, **159** 10, 42–4.

Melia, K. (1980) Saving Life – a difficult decision. *Nursing*, 1st Series **15**, 631–2.

Melia, K. (1987) Everyday ethics for nurses: cruel to be kind? *Nursing Times* (April) 43–5.

Munn, V.A. and Tichy, A.M. (1987) Nurses' perceptions of stressors in pediatric intensive care. *J. Pediatr. Nurs.*, 2 **6**, 405–11.

Pallis, C. (1982) ABC of brain stem death. *Br. Med. J.*, **285**, 1409.

President's Commission for the Study of Ethical Problems in Medicine and Biomedical and Behavioural Research (1983) *Deciding to Forego Life-sustaining treatment*. The Commission, Washington.

Rowden, R. (1987) The extended role of the nurse. *Nursing*, 3rd Series **14**, 516–7.

Rumbold, G. (1986) *Ethics in Nursing Practice*. Baillière Tindall, Eastbourne.

Stinson, P. and Stinson, R. (1983) *The Long Dying of Baby Andrew*, Atlantic Monthly Press.

Stinson, R. and Stinson, P. (1979) On the death of a baby. *J. Med. Ethics*, **7**, 5–18.

Thayer, M.B. (1987) The Nurse Manager: Clarifying Ethical Issues in Professional Role Responsibility. *Pediatr. Nurs.*, **13** (6), 430–2.

Tinker, J. (1978) General intensive therapy. In *Intensive Care*, Nursing Times Publications, London.

Todres, I.D. (1985) Ethical issues in paediatric intensive care. In *Proceedings of the 4th World Congress on Intensive and Critical Care Medicine*. King and Wirth Publishing Co. Ltd, London.

UKCC (1984) *Code of Professional Conduct for the Nurse, Midwife and Health Visitor*. United Kingdom Central Council, London.

Verzemnieks, I.L. and Nash, D. (1984) Ethical issues related to pediatric care. *Nursing Clinics of North America*, **19** (2), 319–28.

Williams, A. (1985) The value of QALYs. *Health and Social Service Journal*.

4

Issues in community care

MARK WHITING

In this chapter, some of the ethical implications arising from the provision of care in the community will be explored. Two main areas of interest require analysis. The first concerns the fundamental matter of the appropriateness or rightness of actively pursuing the philosophy of community based care of children, as opposed to providing that care within the institutional setting. The second part of this chapter will address more specific ethical issues which arise for particular groups of children and with regard to specific aspects of care.

Within the following discussion, it is assumed that the predominant underlying philosophy which runs throughout the health service is that of utilitarianism, i.e. endeavouring to achieve the greatest all round good for all concerned with the care of any individual patient. Many ethical problems which occur within the health-care arena originate in the conflict which arises between this philosophy of utilitarianism, and the ideas embodied within the Hippocratic oath of 'the preservation of life at all costs' and 'the sanctity of human life'. In the text to follow, some aspects of this conflict are explored in detail.

As a general principle, medical morality reflects the morality of wider society; indeed, it could be described as a major subsystem of the current social morality. However, rapid advancement in the health-care domain is such that as new techniques become available through scientific and technological progress, the world of medicine is continually asking questions the answers to which can not be found within our existing social morality (the current debate surrounding the use of living embryo tissue in the treatment of disease provides a particularly good example of this). The philosophy of promoting community care highlights a number of issues generated within the medical world which wider society will be required to address in the very near future.

IS COMMUNITY CARE RIGHT?

The notion of community care is by no means a new idea. Indeed, throughout history the community has always provided the setting in which the great majority of medical and nursing care has been given. Only in the 19th and early 20th centuries has institutional care, as provided by large hospitals, superseded community care in the management of selected illnesses. In the UK, more recently, and throughout the relatively short life of the National Health Service, the hospital sector has concentrated its work largely in the management of acute illness. In addition to this, long-term institutional care has been provided for the elderly and those suffering from problems related to mental health as well as those with mental and physical handicap. During the last ten years in particular, there has been a marked acceleration in the move away from institutional care and toward community care, especially with regard to those client-care groups mentioned above.

This shift has, however, created a great many problems. With particular regard to those suffering from mental handicap, the philosophy of mass de-institutionalization has attracted much criticism. The consequences of actively pursuing the re-introduction to society of large numbers of people who had been the victims of long-term hospitalization, although anticipated well in advance, have not been adequately catered for. The needs of this population were seriously underestimated, and community service provision was inadequate. Questions have therefore been asked about the appropriateness of the community care philosophy. Unless adequate provision is made for care in the community setting, then the practical interpretation of the philosophy may ruin the good intentions behind it. Indeed, the intent underlying the community care ethos is based on the belief that such action is right, and more appropriate than the alternative of hospitalization. The belief remains that it is in the best interest of the long-term institutionalized population that they should move from enormous impersonal institutions, in which they have been housed for many years, into the society from whence they originally came.

The same philosophy of care that has resulted in this mass exodus from the long-stay hospitals has permeated many parts of the health service, and the policy of community care continues to be followed in the belief that it is correct and in the best interest of the patient.

This begs the following questions: Is the philosophy of community care really in the best interest of the individual and of those who will be responsible for meeting his or her needs in the community? Is it in the best interest of wider society? Is the motivation behind the pursuance of the community care ethos truly utilitarian, i.e. for the greatest good of everyone?

In answering these questions, it is necessary to look at the rationale behind the move away from institutional care for those who are ill. The earlier policy of routine hospitalization was deeply embedded in the utilitarian philosophy which, in turn, lay behind the social and political changes in the 19th century, a philosophy which exerted a very positive influence on the development of our present welfare state. It may appear at first glance a little strange to describe both the policy of mass institutionalization and that of deliberate large scale de-institutionalization as being based on the same utilitarian philosophy. However, this apparent anomaly belies much of the fundamental basis of ethical reasoning. The solution to this problem, and indeed the key to the discussion of many ethical questions is to be found in the broader social context within which those ethical questions arise.

This contextual consideration is an essential part of any ethical discussion, although it could be argued that the nature of general social morality is largely fixed. In fact, although broader social policy as determined by government, in it's widest sense, has a certain permanence that can be seen to be founded in the philosophy of beneficence and non-maleficence, it would be inadvisable to view specific ethical problems outside the wider social context within which they are located.

Consider the following. The hospitalization of the sick child in the late 19th and early 20th centuries was often believed by many at the time to be the most appropriate way to manage both acute illness and long-term medical problems. Of course, this was not merely a feature of the relationship between medical and lay society in Victorian England, but was also a reflection of a more general societal attitude to children that was prevalent at this time. A period of ostracism from the family was often seen as being therapeutic for the child, even when he or she was well!

Many Victorian hospitals refused to admit children, although around the time that the Hospital For Sick Children was founded (1852), a period of hospitalization was considered to be an effective therapeutic stratagem in itself. As medical expertise developed apace, and as the precursors of our present welfare state came into being, a paternalistic attitude toward the care of the sick emerged. At that time, it was considered by those responsible for determining social policy that the care of the sick was the exclusive domain of the experts, the medical profession and thus, institutional care became the widely accepted norm.

For many years, to have a child admitted to hospital was to surrender the child to the nursing and medical staff completely. The child admitted to an infectious diseases hospital was abandoned by his parents to white shrouded attendants – ghoulish figures to the fevered imagination of a child – and not rescued again until he was completely recovered which could be a matter of weeks or months according to the degree of complexity of the disease. The only visiting that the child was allowed was if his name appeared on the 'danger list'; when it was unlikely that either the child or his parents would recognise each other.

(Saunders, 1982).

The above quotation demonstrates the extent to which the policy of hospitalization was pursued. Although we might now regard this action as both inappropriately paternalistic and misguided, it was believed at the time that this therapeutic stratagem was in the best interest of the child and in the best interest of all concerned in his or her care. This was a reflection of the utilitarian view that actions should result in the greatest all round happiness (see the work of John Stuart Mill for a detailed exposition of this philosophy). However, this notion was fundamentally flawed. As was evident long before John Bowlby's work on 'Attachment and Loss' in which the theory of maternal deprivation is expounded, 'happiness' is not often to be found in the young child who is removed from his or her parents and home. It is clear, therefore, that for the utilitarian ethos to achieve its goals, it must be based upon demonstrable fact and not just on some tenuous half-truth.

However commendable the intentions of those who would have us believe that a particular action is 'for the best', it is essential that the experts base their expertise on irrefutable fact and not simply on what is believed to be right at that point in time. How many Victorian children suffered from the pain and unhappiness that prolonged hospitalization entailed, solely because at that time the experts believed that hospitalization was not only the key to the conquest of disease, but served the best interest of the child and his or her family?

The processes by which decisions are made are often based upon a fundamentally flawed argument or a 'fact' that is eventually disproved. Even in these supposedly enlightened days, decisions can only be made in the light of the current level of knowledge. It would be inappropriate to enter into a detailed discussion on the nature of knowledge at this point, however the extremes of this debate are to be found in the work on the one hand of Karl Popper and on the other of Thomas Kuhn.

Briefly summarized, Popper sees knowledge as being evolutionary; developing as a result of scientific enquiry, whereas Kuhn describes the development of new knowledge as a cyclical process that is irrevocably embedded in the socially contingent nature of that knowledge. This fundamental debate over the nature of knowledge has major implications for any discussion of ethics. It is clear that the resolution of moral dilemmas relies on the utilization of current knowledge. If this knowledge is ill-founded, and based on anything less than irrefutable fact, decisions may be made which subsequently, with the benefit of hindsight, are considered to have been morally wrong. The example of routinely hospitalizing children whenever minor illness occurred provides a case in point.

By their very nature, moral dilemmas arise because a number of conflicting, possibly mutually exclusive alternatives face those who are to make decisions. Of course, when such decisions are required at short notice, or when no precedent exists, then it may not be possible to call upon all available knowledge in making that decision. However, when solutions are required to more long-term problems, such knowledge can generally be drawn upon, and decisions of an ethical nature can be made in the light of this current level of knowledge.

The removal of sick children from their parents, their families and their homes as was the want of the paternalistic 19th century medical lobby would now be considered by many to be immoral. The work of John Bowlby, James Robertson and others in the investigation of the effects of the separation of young children from their parents resulted in the generation of new knowledge. It is now widely accepted that maternal deprivation and separation can have long-standing deleterious effects upon the mental health of the young child. It is largely due to this work, which prompted a re-thinking in medical attitudes, that the care of sick children has shown a slow but steady move away from the hospital and toward the community.

It is now widely accepted that the mass hospitalization of sick children, for example, in the 19th century infectious disease hospital was wrong. An active policy of promoting community care is now very much the accepted norm, and it seems likely that this policy will develop and move forward as time progresses. But what are the implications of this policy and what ethical questions will arise as it is interpreted into practical action?

It is presently estimated that almost one million children are admitted to hospitals in England and Wales each year (Caring for Children in the Health Services, 1987). This figure has increased steadily since the 1950s, when the adverse psychological effects of hospitalization upon young children first gained widespread recognition. However, there has been a tremendous reduction in the average length of hospital stay for children across a wide range of medical and surgical specialities (OPCS, 1985: the average hospital stay for children 0–14 years of age is 4.9 days). In addition, much more child care is managed on a day case or out-patient basis. Increased consumer awareness and a notable decrease in traditional medical paternalism have seen the development of the role of the parent as a partner in care. The consequences of this for the management of childhood illness are far-reaching.

The ethical issues that are raised by the involvement of lay people in the medical decision-making process are tremendous. With particular reference to the care of children, the implications for all involved in the provision of care must be fully explored. When the lay population are involved, i.e. the parents of a sick child, in making decisions of an ethical nature, it is useful to consider the consequences of accepting that the parents have a valuable contribution to make to such decisions. The ideology that medical expertise is based on sounder knowledge than that of the lay population is a myth that is finally being exploded. The medical conscience does not always know better than the lay conscience which of two possible alternative actions is right, and which is likely to be of greatest benefit for a child and his or her family. However, this need not necessarily give rise to conflict, and it is only occasionally that parents and professionals will take opposing views when ethical problems arise. This is of particular relevance in respect of the issues which might arise from a discussion concerning the most appropriate site in which to provide care, i.e. hospital or community. Consider the following hypothetical example:

Stephen, aged seven, is dying in hospital, and his parents desperately want to take him home so that he can die in the house he has lived in since birth rather than in an institution he has known for only a few short weeks. The hospital medical staff are reluctant to discharge Stephen into the community, because they feel that support services will be inadequate and that an intolerable burden will be placed upon his parents if they take Stephen home.

Although all concerned would act only in the child's best interest, the problems which arise from the opposing views that are held by those concerned with his care are unlikely to be rapidly resolved. This in itself will significantly affect his progress.

In discussing the shift from hospital to community care, other factors must, however, be considered. It has long been maintained that community care can provide a substantially cheaper alternative to hospital care. It may well be that future health strategies will begin to exploit this belief more fully. Hospital resources are, after all, finite and when such resources are stretched, early discharge or selective admission policies may reduce some of the strain within the hospital setting. A more sinister motive behind the pursuance of the community care philosophy can therefore arise from the simple economic reality that hospital care, which is becoming increasingly sophisticated and more expensive, may be a cost that society at large is no longer prepared to pay.

While the philosophy of community care is considered to be of benefit to the child and family (particularly with regard to the psychological well-being of the child), and is believed to be less burdensome on society as a whole (in purely financial terms), community care provides us with an option that all would see as desirable. However, if circumstances were such that the needs of the child and family were in conflict with the demands of wider society – for instance if the parents of a sick child expressed extreme discomfort at the prospect of providing care in their own home – how far would it be reasonable and justifiable for pressure to be exerted by the hospital staff to secure discharge? Would it be fair for medical and nursing staff to attempt to force the parents to take the child home?

Those nurses and doctors who are responsible for the interpretation and implementation of the philosophy of redirecting care away from the hospital and toward the community must be sure not to lose sight of the principles of benevolence and respect for the child and his or her family which should take precedence over all other considerations.

Hopefully, the foregoing discussion has introduced some of the fundamental issues that will arise as the philosophy of community care continues to be pursued in the future. In the second part of this chapter, more specific issues will be explored, drawing on some of the principles and ideas that have been introduced above.

ETHICAL ISSUES IN COMMUNITY CARE

As mentioned previously, contextual considerations have a very important part to play when discussing ethical issues. In the earlier example, the contextual parameter of time was highlighted. In the remainder of this chapter, the parameter of location will form the basis for discussion. In this particular case, the location is the community, to be more precise, the home in which a child with specific health related needs is to be cared for.

A number of specific, hypothetical scenarios will be introduced to illustrate some of the many ethical issues which may arise as the move away from hospital and toward community care progresses.

Decision-making

When a child is admitted to hospital, many of those responsibilities which are normally fulfilled by his or her parents are removed from them. Despite the good intentions of enlightened nurses and doctors who may endeavour to normalize hospital life, and regardless of staff commitment to parental participation in care, it remains extremely difficult to accommodate all the wishes of parents in retaining control of their child's daily life while in hospital. It is inevitable that parents will give up many aspects of the role that they have previously maintained for their child throughout his or her life.

When a child is cared for at home, however, parental control and responsibility are generally preserved. Decisions are made by parents with regard to all aspects of a child's daily living. This applies equally to decisions concerning specific health-care needs, such as administering oxygen to a child with cystic fibrosis, as it does to any other aspect of the child's care, for example deciding at what time to take the child to bed.

Of course, parents have always had such responsibilities, and it is correct that they should make decisions about their child's care. Why then is this responsibility removed from parents as soon as their child is admitted to hospital? The only reasonable justification that could be made is that parents do not have the specific knowledge and expertise that is required to deal with discrete health-related problems. Of course, in many instances, this is indeed true, however it must be acknowledged that the very act of hospitalization does not immediately disable parents from making decisions about aspects of care which would be constant regardless of the child's medical conditions. Additionally, it is clear that with time, parents can be equipped with information and skills that will allow them to play a crucial role in even the most complicated and technical aspects of care.

It is essential that once a child is discharged from hospital, or alternatively, if his or her parents are offered the option to care for him or her at home throughout his or her illness, health-care professionals must endeavour to impart the necessary knowledge and skill that will allow parents to acquire sufficient expertise to deal with any problems that may arise. No matter how much support may be given to the family, and regardless of how much time nurses and doctors are able to give to them in their own homes, the fact remains that parents will often be left alone. They will have to make decisions that will affect their child's health, even to the extent of determining whether the child may live or die. As the so-called experts in health related problems, we must strive to ensure that we meet the parental need to share in knowledge that previous generations of nurses and doctors have striven to shroud in mystery.

It must be accepted by the nursing and medical professions that to attempt to withhold such knowledge from the lay population is wrong, and may, in fact, be construed as professional negligence. The idea of protecting parents by withholding any information which may assist them when making decisions concerning their child's care reflects a paternalistic attitude which we would do well to reject once and for all.

The reasons why paternalism, albeit in the name of protecting the patient, has survived are deeply embedded in the culture of Western society. In the recent past, however, as the consumerist movement has spread into the health-care arena, medical paternalism has begun to give way to an acceptance that both lay society as a whole, and in particular patients and their relatives have an increasing role to play in medical decision-making.

The significance of this for the child being nursed at home is considerable. Decisions which may previously have been made by doctors alone, are increasingly being made by patients, their families and the whole health-care team. When decisions are fairly straight-forward, this team effort is clearly a very positive development. However, if conflicts arise, because differing opinions are held by those involved in care, then the ethical implications may be consider-able. This is of particular significance in the home situation, where parental opinions are most likely to be strongly voiced. As social anthropologists would acknowledge, man is a territorial animal, at his strongest and most determined when on home ground. In the home situation, parents are therefore more likely to want their point of view to be both heard and accepted. Consider the following examples:

Stephanie, a five year old girl, has chronic liver and kidney failure, and after a protracted period of illness in hospital, has been discharged home to die. Her parents, who have previously accepted the inevitability of Stephanie's death, are giving mild pain killers and withholding stronger opiate analgesia in the hope that her time at home with them will be lengthened. The home nurse and GP who were closely involved in the decision to send Stephanie home realize that she is in pain, but are unable to persuade her parents to give more powerful analgesia.

Daniel, aged eight, has an inoperable cerebral tumour. His parents are nursing him at home. He has only a short time to live. The family GP visits and find that Daniel is deeply asleep. He stays and talks with the family for some time, and Daniel begins to wake. The GP observes Daniel's mother giving him some oral morphine. Mother explains that she administers pain relief each time he wakes, because she believes he is in pain. Despite the GP's insistence that Daniel does not need to be given so much analgesia, both parents insist that this is the only way to keep him pain free.

In the circumstances presented above, who is right, and who is wrong? The parents of both children feel that they are doing what is best for their child. What are the implications for professional nurses and doctors who are presented with such difficult dilemmas?

Surely the greatest wrong of all would be to suggest that responsibility should be completely taken away from parents in such situations.

Of course, this again raises the fundamental matter of whether the consciences of medical and nursing staff know better than the consciences of parents in such situations. Is it fair to pressurize parents into accepting the supposedly more objective views of nurses and doctors? Is it right that parents should be denied the freedom of choice? Is it just to impose medical morality upon them in such situations?

There are no easy answers to such questions. The problem is one that members of the nursing and medical professions must be prepared to address as we strive to involve the parents in decision-making. In the majority of situations, where there is little difficulty in reaching a decision that is acceptable to all, this will not cause problems. However, when a number of alternative options presents us with a choice, professional carers must be prepared to listen to and accept the opinions of those most intimately involved in the child's care.

The dying child

Although many child deaths are unpredictable, for example, the consequence of acute illness or as a result of an accident, large numbers of deaths in childhood can be foreseen well in advance. This includes those children dying as a result of congenital problems such as cardiac abnormality, those with inherited diseases, for example cystic fibrosis, and those with acquired conditions such as leukaemia.

For these children and their families, where medical care will not produce a cure, and death is inevitable, the option of community care, and the possibility of the child dying at home is one that is increasingly becoming available. Professional carers have long recognized that hospitals can be rather impersonal. Despite the efforts of enlightened nurses and doctors who may endeavour to create a friendly and caring environment in hospital, for the young child it is unlikely to prove an adequate substitute for the security, warmth and love that he or she may remember as 'home'. The introduction of hospice care facilities, although still fairly sparse in the UK, provides a valuable alternative to the busy acute children's ward. However, for the majority of children, the choice is limited to either the acute paediatric ward or his or her home. In certain circumstances, for a variety of reasons, there may be no choice at all, and the option of home care may not be offered to the family, or in some situations, may be totally impractical. Indeed, some parents may consider the idea of their child dying at home to be abhorrent.

As professionals, it is essential that we are sensitive to the wishes of the parents and, of course, to the wishes of the child. Wherever it is possible to consider a number of options, whenever time is available to discuss all possible alternatives with the family, and, where appropriate, the child, every effort should be made to respect the views of the family. It would be wrong to coerce unwilling parents into taking their dying child home, whatever the reasons for the parents' reluctance may be. It would equally be wrong to deny the parents the option of home care if that was their wish. The following examples may highlight some of the issues to be overcome:

Sonia, aged seven, has leukaemia. Despite intensive chemotherapy and radiotherapy, she has recently relapsed. Her parents are told that no curative medical intervention is now possible and that Sonia has only a short time to live. Throughout her protracted illness, Sonia's parents have required intense psychological support. Each new crisis has given rise to almost overwhelming distress. The nursing and medical staff feel that the parents would put themselves under extreme pressure if they were to take Sonia home to die. The family live in a secluded rural village where community medical and nursing support is thought to be somewhat limited. The extended families of both parents live many miles away. Sonia is unaware of her prognosis but wants to go home. Sonia's parents say that they feel they should take her home, but each time practical arrangements to transfer her home are discussed, both appear highly stressed. How should the situation be handled?

Anita, aged ten months, has an inoperable congenital cardiac defect. Although she has been admitted to hospital a number of times with respiratory tract infections, she has predominantly been looked after at home by her mother, with support from the Community Paediatric Nurses, based at the local hospital, and her GP. As winter approaches, she suffers a series of acute respiratory tract infections requiring hospital treatment, and her cardiac status deteriorates. Her parents are told that Anita will probably not survive the winter, and are offered the opportunity to take her home. The parents refuse, saying that they do not feel able to cope with her prognosis. Mother who has been resident with Anita decides that she no longer wishes to stay with her. Parental visiting becomes less frequent. How should the situation be handled?

David, aged six, has end-stage renal failure. His parents have been told that he cannot be cured, and they have decided that they wish to take him home to die. Much of David's treatment has been painful, disruptive and distressing for his family. David has an older brother and sister who haven't seen him at home for almost a year. They are aware that David will not survive. Arrangements have been made for community support services to be laid on as soon as the family arrive home. As David is about to be discharged home to die, the hospital medical staff are made aware of an innovative treatment that might possibly prolong his life, however it is likely to have devastating physical and pysiological effects upon him and may in fact kill him. How should the situation be handled?

Discussion of issues surrounding death and its management raise many ethical questions for those professionals who are involved in the provision of care for children who are dying. There are no ready made answers.

The responsibilities of nurses and doctors are basically two-fold. First, all possible information regarding treatment and facilities available to the child must be openly explored. Secondly, professionals must be highly sensitive to the needs and wishes of the child and his or her parents, and should endeavour to avoid the imposition of their own morality and values upon the family.

Technological advancement?

As medical and scientific technology has developed in the recent past, our ability to save life has expanded enormously. The particular consequences of this in the management of premature birth, and of the child who is critically ill, have given rise to a whole series of new moral dilemmas. By the provision of intensive medical and nursing care, many children and babies are recovered from the brink of death, and, following a period of intensive intervention and all-out system support, many children's lives can be saved. For those who make a full recovery with no residual handicap, the justification for this intensive care is unquestionable, however, when the outcome is rather less favourable, when gross mental or physical damage persists, the morality or rightness of the decisions to provide such care may be questioned. Of particular concern are the consequences for the parents of such children, who inevitably will be expected to take on the responsibility for providing long-term care.

Historically, many such children as well as those with congenital and inherited handicap have lived out their lives in large institutions, however, nowadays the great majority of such children will be looked after at home by their parents and families. This raises a number of ethical questions. Consider the following:

Michelle, aged 15, is pregnant; she has successfully concealed her pregnancy from family and friends. She goes into spontaneous labour and delivers a baby whose estimated gestational age is 23 weeks. The baby is nursed on a neonatal intensive care unit where he is ventilated. The baby suffers a number of intra-ventricular haemorrhages and also several prolonged bradycardiac episodes. The baby gains weight, and appears to be growing steadily. Despite obvious neurological impairment, he is weaned from the ventilator at 11 weeks of age. The baby, now named Robert by his mother, seems to be making satisfactory progress, but suffers a respiratory and then cardiac arrest. He is resuscitated following a prolonged period of asystole, and requires further resuscitation several times before being finally weaned from the ventilator at 18 weeks. Michelle has managed to visit most days, her parents have been largely unsupportive, her boyfriend deserted her when Robert was born, and she is still attending school. Robert has a pronounced neurological deficit and is possibly blind. Michelle says that she loves and wants the baby, but feels she will not be able to cope when she is discharged home. Strenuous efforts by Social Services and community health care staff fail to produce any support from Michelle's family, who are refusing to allow Michelle to bring Robert into the family home. He is still in hospital several weeks after being pronounced 'fit for discharge'.

Jenny, aged seven, has been involved in a road traffic accident, and has sustained a fractured skull and cervical spinal damage. A brain scan identifies a large sub-arachnoid haemorrhage. She undergoes emergency neurological surgery. During a long stay on the intensive care unit, she remains unstable and requires repeated cardio-pulmonary resuscitation. Some days later, her intra-cranial pressure is noted to be rising, and further neurosurgery is considered necessary. Jenny has remained unconscious throughout this time. Jenny's parents feel reluctant to consent to further surgery, they feel that she has already suffered so much, but are persuaded when told that she will die without it. Jenny's operation relieves the intra-cranial pressure, but she remains in coma. Family and friends are with Jenny almost continually, she shows no response, but is able to breathe spontaneously. Six months after the accident, Jenny's condition has shown no change, she remains totally reliant upon nursing care. The possibility of discharge is to be discussed with Jenny's parents who have both returned to full-time employment in the family business.

Although these examples are perhaps a little extreme, the issues raised by the questions of resuscitation and the provision of intensive care are very real. They are faced every day by nurses and doctors, who, in emergency situations are required to make decisions whose long-term consequences are largely unpredictable, but potentially devastating. As our ability to preserve life becomes ever greater, the ethical implications of decisions which are made in such situations will continue to give rise to moral dilemmas.

The child

It is perhaps fitting to return in this final section to the role of the child in dealing with problems of an ethical nature. It is, after all, the child who is the subject of this whole book.

From the moment a child is born, he or she begins to play an ever increasing role in the decision-making processes surrounding his or her life. In the early days this is manifested principally in terms of very practical aspects of daily living (for example, protestation at certain tastes or sensations), but as the child grows older, he or she begins to participate in increasingly more complex decisions. Of course parental protection is absolute during the early years of life, however, as the child grows and matures, most parents begin to involve their children in many aspects of decision making. Even before the age when a child is able to present a coherent argument in favour of a particular point of view, the parents will be aware of his or her wishes and needs and will strive to incorporate them into their own opinions. The growing child will be able to verbalize his or her own opinions at a very early age, and as he or she becomes more independent his or her need to be involved in decisions of an increasingly abstract nature, including those related to ethical problems will invariably increase.

However complicated a particular problem may be, and however painful a particular experience may prove, every effort must be made to ensure that the child is involved, wherever possible, in decisions which are to affect his or her life (or death).

When all is said and done, it is principally through our recognition that children themselves seek the security, warmth and love of their own home that we have moved inexorably toward the community as the most appropriate site for the management of much childhood illness.

Whenever complex or difficult problems are to be confronted, it is the responsibility of all professionals who are in any way involved in the care of a child to ensure that every consideration is given to the wishes of that child and those of his or her parents.

REFERENCES

Bowlby, J. (1951) *Maternal Care and Mental Health.* World Health Organisation, Geneva.

Caring for Children in the Health Service (1987) *Where are the Children?* NAWCH, London.

Kuhn, T. (1962) *The Structure of Scientific Resolution.* 2nd edn, University of Chicago Press, Chicago.

Mill, J.S. (1867) *Utilitarianism.* 3rd edn, Longman's, London.

OPCS (1985) *Hospital In-Patient Enquiry, 1983.*

Popper, K. (1975) *Objective Knowledge.* Routledge and Kegan Paul, London.

Robertson, J. (1958) *Young Children in Hospital.* Tavistock, London.

Saunders, D.M. (1982) *Sick Children's Nursing.* In Allen, P. and Jolley, M. *Nursing, Midwifery and Health Visiting since 1900.* Faber & Faber, London.

FURTHER READING

Campbell, A.V. (1984) *Moral Dilemmas in Medicine.* Churchill Livingstone, New York.

5

Ethical issues in the practise of nursing in child psychiatry: an overview based on an interactionist model

WALLACE B. HAMILTON

A detailed search of the literature in preparation for this chapter, including that of a bibliography of British publications on nursing in child, adolescent and family psychiatry (Hamilton, 1988), failed to bring to light any material concerned with the ethical issues involved in the practise of nursing in child psychiatry.

To provide a systematic base for an overview of the topic, this chapter will offer an interactionist model for nursing in this specialized field of psychiatric care. Thereafter an attempt will be made to identify and briefly examine some of the fundamental (everyday) ethical issues in child psychiatric nursing. The chapter will conclude with brief comments on some of the implications for nurse education and training.

AN INTERACTIONIST MODEL FOR NUSING

The theory of an interactionist model for the interpersonal behaviour of one-to-one and group experiences suggests that the people involved are interactive agents, who are inseparably linked with, and in turn influenced by, their perceptions of each other and of the environment in which their behaviour is performed.

This theoretical basis can be applied with reasonable ease to nurse(s)–child(ren) interactions in day and residential settings for emotionally disturbed children. Within the parameters of a one-to-one relationship the nurse and child can be understood not only as each having a perception of the other and interacting as one person to another, but also as each having a uniquely personal perception of the environment with which they are concurrently interacting. Additionally, they will share what is a collective perception of the environment and as a two person unit will be interacting with that. Where the one-to-one relationship is taking place within the space of a group then that two person unit must open its parameters to include their uniquely personal and collective perceptions of, and their interactions with, the population of the group and its environment.

THE PRACTISE OF NURSING IN CHILD PSYCHIATRY

The growing demands from both inside and outside the profession for the development of extensions to the role of nurses, and with these the need for them to assume greater degrees of accountability and responsibility, have made it a matter of some priority that the practise of nursing be better defined than it is at the moment.

However, the task of definition is not as easy as first impressions might suggest. There are areas of health-care where the boundaries of practise between nursing and that of other health-care professionals are intentionally not at all clear cut. One such area is child psychiatry. On admission to a day or residential unit the child (and family) will be cared for by a multi-disciplinary team. Whilst much will depend on how a unit defines its functions as a multi-disciplinary facility, there will inevitably be elements of clarity and diffusion surrounding the roles of the professions involved.

Within that kind of working space the nurses will be constantly confronted with fundamental ethical issues. Using the interactionist model, it can be concluded that some of these issues will be unique to the nurse(s), some to the nurse(s)–child(ren)–environment interactions, while others will arise only within the context of the clarity and diffusion of multi-disciplinary roles.

The fundamental ethical issues can be overviewed within the process of compiling a nursing history, formulating a nursing diagnosis, prescribing nursing care, providing the care and judging the effectiveness of care.

Compiling a nursing history

If nurses are to practise to the highest possible professional standards it is essential that they should know as much about the child and family as is required for the effective assessment, planning, implementation and evaluation of nursing care. The compiling of a nursing history provides a systematic approach to getting that information, which must have something to say not only about the child's current lifestyle but also about what that was like before the onset of his or her problems. At first glance the compilation of a nursing history appears to be a laudable and straightforward ideal. However, a somewhat closer look will demonstrate that it is open to some fundamental ethical issues.

One of the issues which needs to be addressed is the nature of the differentiation between the content of a nursing history and one which has been compiled for a medical purpose. Traditionally the nursing literature has offered the explanation that a nursing history is concerned with the effects of an illness on the patient and his or her family, while a medical history is concerned only with the illness itself. Apart from the criticism that this definition implies that members of the medical profession are not expected to be interested in patients and families as people – and is thereby open to the charge that it is nothing more than a value judgement of very questionable quality – how useful is it anyway in a multi-disciplinary health-care setting with its clarity and diffusion of roles, and where in any case the concept of illness may not be one which is readily accepted.

If it can be reasonably granted that in a child psychiatric setting, at least, the traditional approach to the content of a nursing history is open to question, then it is clear that the matter is one for examination. For example, some important questions need to be asked about who decides what information is required for the practise of nursing, and thereafter what is the specific nature of the information which nurses need. It is very tempting to advocate the totality of the strict approach that all matters of direct nursing care are for nurses, and that it is they alone who should determine what information is needed for their practise. However, there is the question as to the validity of the argument that such an absolute is probably not a very helpful one in the context of the multi-disciplinary provision of health-care and its inherent inter-professional relationships. Indeed, nurses might also consider the validity of the argument that neither does it augur well for the best interests of the child and family.

Perhaps though, the basic intention of that approach can be more clearly and helpfully expressed. The issue may be capable of being better understood if it were viewed as being not so much one of the questioning acceptance or denial of the totality of an absolute, but rather as one which was seeking to promote an examination of the extent to which a group of nurses were able to clarify their role(s) in a multi-disciplinary health-care setting. Given that new perspective, would nurses then be any better placed to determine a rationale within which the intention of the nursing for nurses approach could be viewed as a perfectly reasonable one to adopt?

If, for the purpose of this overview, it can now be assumed that it is possible for a group of nurses to determine the elements of clarity in the role(s) they fulfil, then who among them bears the responsibility for deciding the nature of the information needed to satisfy the role(s)? It would appear to be logical to suggest that only those nurses who had a Registered education and training should attempt to determine the contents of a nursing history. After all is it not them on whom the professional responsibility and account-ability rests for the standard of care provided. This would advocate that it is the Sister(s)/Charge Nurse(s), then the Staff Nurse(s), who should determine what information about a child and family is needed for the effective provision of nursing care. However, to what extent can it be argued that a logical response and an ethical one are one and the same? A number of day and residential wards and units will have a nursing group which is by no means entirely made up of Registered Nurses. For example, in some groups Nursery Nurses will form a substantial numerical proportion of the nursing establishment. Their skills lie particularly in the area of play activities, and they may have play skills which generously exceeed those of a Registered Nurse. Indeed, in any event, irrespective of educational training and experience background, it would be quite unrealistic to expect every individual in a given group of nurses to possess the same range of personal qualities and nursing skills. Inevitably, within the overall nursing group, there will be collectively a wide range of qualities and skills available for the appropriate nursing care of the varying situations which arise in a child psychiatric setting. Whilst it may be granted that on the grounds of professional accountability and responsibility it is the Registered

Nurse who determines the quality of care to be provided, the issue nevertheless remains as to what extent – and in what manner – should they discuss the contents of a nursing history with other nurses and allow themselves to be influenced by what they say they need to know about a child if they are to fulfil their designated role(s)?

When, thereafter, they are determining the nature of the specific content of a nursing history the nurses must examine very carefully the need to maintain the individuality (or the totality) of each child. Given that each child is a unique human being, a fundamental issue here is one of determining how far should nurses go towards having a universal and pre-determined proforma for the compilation of data. It can be easily granted that some of the required details about each child will be so similar that a measure of pre-determination will not be entirely out of place. It remains important, however, that nurses decide the extent to which a proforma will determine the specificity of the information which is to be compiled, and the extent to which the nature of the specificity will be left to the clinical judgement of the nurse who is conducting the compilation of the history.

No matter who among the nurses asks the questions of the child and family, and who will thereafter compile a nursing history from the answers supplied, the matter of confidentiality of information looms large. Two aspects appear to need attention. On the one hand there is the degree to which any item of information is confidential to the interaction between the child, the family and the one nurse who is compiling the history, and on the other the degree to which the information which finally appears in the history is confidential to the extended interaction between the child, the family and the nursing group, and then beyond that to the members of the multi-disciplinary team. Clearly each child and family has the unchallengeable right to expect that the rules of confidentiality will be maintained. Such rules are not always clear cut. In exercising their obligations to both child and family and to the need to uphold standards of professional conduct, nurses must constantly use their individual judgement to achieve an acceptable balance between the need to keep the information confidential to the purpose for which it was given (i.e. in this case the child's nursing care), and the degree to which it can be assumed that both child and family know and understand that the information provided may in some circumstances be beneficially and properly made available to the members of the other disciplines who are involved in the delivery of their total health-care (United Kingdom Central Council for Nursing, Midwifery and Health Visiting, 1984, 1987a,b).

A nursing history can reasonably be described as the foundation upon which the effective practise of nursing skills rests. It is therefore of some importance that every step is taken to ensure that its compilation is undertaken in a manner which is as professionally correct as possible. Only by nurses asking questions about their practise which are seemingly of an everyday nature, but about which there are so often no ready answers, can the right start ever be achieved.

Formulating a nursing diagnosis

In this stage of the practise of nursing it is the task of the practitioner(s) to use clinical judgement to identify and describe, from the information provided in a nursing history, those needs and problems of a particular child which may be considered the most likely to respond to nursing care. This process can be correctly called the formulation of a nursing diagnosis.

Many practitioners of nursing, either as individuals or as a member of a group, will be carrying out a process not unlike that as part of their professional responsibilities, development and as an extension of their role(s). A major issue, however, is centred around the dichotomy between what nurses say they are practising and what they are perceived by others as actually doing.

An important function of a diagnosis is that of promoting a means of effective communication among, at least, the set of professionals for whom it is intended. Clearly, then, the diagnoses which are formulated must be based on a scheme of classification and a glossary, each having a demonstrable theoretical basis capable of being unambiguously understood by each member; although the nursing profession in Britain has not as yet developed a scheme for classification nor a glossary for nursing diagnosis. While it may be viewed as a matter of some urgency that nurses in Britain do have some uniform understanding for the identification and description of children's needs and problems, it is an easier thing to say (or write) than to achieve.

No matter at what stage in the development of a process for the formulation of a nursing diagnosis the profession happens to be at and whatever form of words a nursing diagnosis might finally take, there are two principles which probably ought to be of concern to the pioneering practitioners. First, the data which the diagnosis provides must have something to say to nurses about the degree of clarity to which a child's needs and problems have been identified and described. Furthermore, the data must indicate the frequency with which each need and problem is presented in the behavioural reper-toire of a child who is emotionally disturbed. Secondly, a nursing diagnosis must provide the practitioner(s) with some indication as to whether the satisfaction of a need or the resolution of a problem needs no nursing intervention whatsoever, needs a minimum level of nursing care, or whether the satisfaction or resolution will be achieved only after a significant input of nursing expertise.

Nowadays a great deal of emphasis is placed on the expectation that nurses will exercise a wholly objective approach to the assess-ment, planning, implementation and evaluation of their care. However, as with many aspects of the behaviour of humans, the helpfulness (or otherwise) of the extremes and excessiveness of their conduct needs to be carefully examined. One of the rationales for the element of objectivity, that nurses are professionally obliged to avoid unhelpful over-attachment and over-protectiveness towards a patient, can be easily appreciated. But in all fairness it must be stated that the degree to which objectivity can be considered to be the only therapeutic approach in the practise of psychiatric nursing care is something which ought to be the focus of critical examina-tion. For example, within the interactionist model offered for this overview (which proposes that in one-to-one and group experiences the behaviour of one person, and by implication his or her delibera-tions and decisions, is influenced by his or her perception of the other and the environment) to what extent can it reasonably be stated that objectivity is the only order of the day?

Perhaps, then, the crux of this difficult matter lies in having a fresh look at the too often unquestioned assumption that objectivity is the hallmark of nurses' professionalism, whereas subjectivity is that of a course of action which is never in the best interest of the patient. If this is the case, then can it be reasonably argued that what is needed is a new rationale for the practise of nursing, which will not so much favour the totality of either objectivity or subjectivity, but will rather seek to clarify the degree to which these elements can be better therapeutically balanced?

What are the implications of this for the formulation of a nursing diagnosis in child psychiatry? We have seen that in the process of formulating a nursing diagnosis the nurses are seeking to be as clear as they can about the nature of a child's needs and problems, the frequency of their presentation and the level of nursing input which will be required for their satisfaction or resolution. If this process is to take place within an interactional experience, to what extent does it follow that a nursing diagnosis is something which should be neither totally objective nor totally subjective in what it has to say to the practitioner? In seeking, then, to achieve a nursing diagnosis which is more balanced between these extremes, to what degree can the practitioner(s) now consider themselves to be professionally obliged to allow factors like subjective feelings, value judgements, inferences and intuition and personal opinion to influence the course of their diagnostic deliberations and decisions?

If the practise of nursing in child psychiatry can lay claim to be child/family-centred then quite clearly the formulation of a nursing diagnosis cannot be left at this point. If practitioners can now at least begin to consider that the diagnostic process is indeed something which is essentially a part of an interaction between the carer and the cared for, then what are the roles of the child and family in the identification and description of needs and problems? If it can be granted that at least some children have roles to fulfil in the formulation of a nursing diagnosis, then what are the emotional, social and intellectual criteria against which an individual child can be judged as able to understand the process and contribute to the deliberations and decisions which need to be made? In so far as the child's parents are concerned, are their particular styles of care (like those of over-protectiveness, over-demanding, oppressive or smothering) something which nurses should be considering when deciding whether or not a particular set of parents can be judged with reason as having very little, or even nothing, to contribute to the formulation of a nursing diagnosis?

Nurses are frequently conscious of the criticism that a medical diagnosis is but a label, which when used can have a very damaging effect on the humanness of the patient to whom it has been applied. Indeed, how often have nurses used the spirit of that criticism for their own ends? If, then, that criticism can be levelled against a medical diagnosis, to what extent can it be used as a criticism against a nursing diagnosis? In seeking to establish the legitimacy of a nursing diagnosis, are nurses not just simply abandoning one type of label in favour of one of their own?

The current state of the art in nursing seems to suggest that there are members of the nursing profession who are indeed very capable of formulating an identification and description of the needs and problems of a particular child. However, if such nursing diagnoses were to be put to the ultimate test and an attempt was made to communicate these to practitioners of nursing having no previous knowledge of the children concerned, to what extent could the outcome be more than intelligently guessed?

For the time being, one of the ethical issues for nurses must be that of the degree to which they can claim that what they are doing can rightly be called the formulation of a nursing diagnosis.

Prescribing nursing care

In so far as this overview is concerned, the nursing care which is required for the satisfaction of a need or the resolution of a problem lies somewhere within a very wide spectrum of physical and psychosocial strategies. It would be most unlikely if, from that range, only one strategy could be identified for the satisfaction or resolution of a particular need or problem. In practise what is much more likely is that for each need/problem two, three or more strategies can be identified. The dual processes of deciding which one can be reasonably considered the most likely to promote the best interests of the child, and its subsequent written inclusion in a nursing care plan, can be referred to as prescribing nursing care. However, before that strategy can be decided upon, let alone written into a care plan, there are some issues which should be addressed.

For children whose behaviour is characterized by features such as muddle, confusion, feelings of uncertainty and lack of confidence the emotional climate of the care setting should be one which is safe, supportive and caring. Factors like the interior design and physical structure of a setting undoubtedly exert important influences on the climate, but it is on the nurses' level of emotional maturity upon which the overall therapeutic ambience (the milieu experience) is founded and developed. The nurses who are professionally responsible and accountable for prescribing nursing care have, then, the very difficult task of determining what are the desirable design and structural features of a care setting (the place) and the nature of the nurses' emotional maturity (the people), then balancing these against the realities of what is available. Ethical dilemmas loom large when decisions have to be made about the criteria against which the desirable features of the place and the emotional maturity of the people should, first, be formulated, and the realities latterly judged. It is on the bases of these realities that final judgements have to be made as to what nursing strategies the place and the people are able to provide in the best interests of the child and family.

Of course very little in the way of nursing care can be prescribed without an adequate range of material and manpower resources being available in, or to, a care setting. Nurses cannot reasonably be expected to provide, say, activity-based experiences for children if they are, for example, any deficiencies in the quality or quantity of equipment, or an insufficient number of capable nurses to make it happen. But questions must be asked about who decides the adequacy or otherwise of a range of equipment (to what extent does it being nice to have a certain toy for the children make that toy a necessary item of equipment for the practise of nursing), what is the optimum number of nurses needed in a particular unit (with what frequency is that number grossly under- or over-estimated), who decides these matters and against what criteria can their decisions be based?

Nurses, rightly, have placed a lot of emphasis on the need to use their collective skills, the unit's climate and the available material and manpower resources to help promote the best interests of the child and family. But the practicalities of nursing are often such that ideals like that are not always very easily achieved. What if, then, the influence exerted by one (or indeed all) of these factors was such that it was too frequently proving to be disadvantageous, resulting in nurses judging that what they were able to provide was not so much their first choice of nursing strategy, but a poor second or even third? Faced with a broad scenario like that, nurses have to decide the specific circumstances in which they would be justified in adopting the role of patient-advocate, then exercising every effort to obtain what they judged they needed for the practise of nursing care, even if that meant disagreeing with the authority of a hospital administration. On the other hand, though, can any specific circumstances be imagined whereby it would be appropriate for nurses to recognize not only the authority of a hospital administration (and incidentally their employee loyalty to it), but additionally the reality of financial and other restraints within which it is obliged to function? This would of course mean nurses adopting a bureaucratic model of practise, to ensure that the order of the hospital administration was maintained. To what extent, though, would this result in nurses having to do what they are already so good at – making do with what they have?

What has not yet been asked, however, is the extent, if any, to which each individual child has a right to contribute to the decisions as to what are his or her best interests. Within the nurse–child parameters of this overview's interactional model, it would seem to be an entirely logical conclusion that each child has some rights in this matter. Some assessment would probably be wise as to the stage of his or her intellectual and moral development and the effects of emotional disturbance on these, not so much for the purpose of determining whether or not the right should be granted in the first place but to promote the judgement about the degree to which the right might be therapeutically exercised. What, too, of the parents' rights to have a say in determining the best interests of their child? The admission of their child to hospital does not normally mean a surrender of parental rights. So, what opportunities to promote the best interests of the child might be lost if the parents are not afforded consultation prior to final decisions being made about which nursing strategy to prescribe?

Nurses also have to keep in mind the fact that whatever strategies they finally select for their nursing care plan have to be capable of being integrated with the care strategies being implemented by the other members of the multi-disciplinary team. To what extent, then, should the practitioners of nursing allow their decisions to be influenced by what other professionals are doing?

Whilst the best interest of the child is a seemingly grand ideal and therefore one which ought to be pursued as forcefully as possible, nurses must always have in mind that each child is nevertheless only one member of a group of children. What, then, of the best interest of the group? Can there ever be any instances whereby it would be reasonable to prescribe nursing strategies which are for the collective good of the group? If this can be granted, then nurses must determine the issues involved in recognizing the circumstances where the best interest of an individual child just simply cannot be given priority over the best interest of the group.

In deciding what strategies of nursing will promote a child's best interests, the practitioner is professionally obliged to give full consideration to the 'Law of Beneficence' (i.e. the right of the carer to determine what is best for the cared for). Nurses must ensure that no act of omission in their practise is detrimental to the welfare of the patient (United Kingdom Central Council for Nursing, Midwifery and Health Visiting 1984). However, in the absence of any specific criteria against which their practise can be judged consistently, nurses must constantly evaluate and define the circumstances in which it can be appropriate to deem that their education, training and experience has demonstrated it is necessary for them to make decisions about the care they should provide, without consultation with others, be they patients, parents or professional colleagues.

The prescribing of nursing care, involving as it does decisions which will influence the lives of a number of people, cannot be taken too lightly. Some of the everyday ethical issues are perhaps deceptively simple, and for that reason are probably all too easily forgotten. No matter how such questions are viewed, to what extent should nurses allow the answers to influence their final selection of nursing strategies?

Providing nursing care

The delivery of nursing care can be quite properly viewed as an area of practise which requires careful consideration and effective decision-making skills.

Whilst most nurses readily agree that the history, diagnosis and prescription are all aspects of what they do, many will take the view that the real work of nurses lies only in the doing of care (i.e. the actual bedside delivery of care).

This point opens the overview to the issues which arise from the dichotomy between being a good practical nurse (i.e. a good doer) and the demands of professional accountability and responsibility where the practitioner should additionally know why specific actions are being taken [i.e. a knowledgeable doer (United Kingdom Central Council for Nursing, Midwifery and Health Visiting 1984, 1986)]. The concepts of a good doer and a knowledgeable one are somewhat tentatively defined in the literature. Is it, for example, sufficient to define a good doer as one who is able (perhaps in doing what comes naturally) to provide for each child's activities of living? If so, and a good standard of practical care is something which can be adequately provided by someone who does not necessarily need a knowledge base, then to what extent can it be argued that the carer need not be a qualified one in the first place? On the other hand, of what possible benefit to a child is a nurse who is knowledgeable in the theory of care but quite inadequate in the area of practical skills? If it can be reasonably granted that neither an unqualified doer nor an unskilled theorist are acceptable personnel for the delivery of care, what of a knowledgeable doer, and how can that concept be defined to its best advantage? In child psychiatry, for instance, no matter whether the delivery of care is being practised within a one-to-one or group interaction, is it sufficient to say that a knowledgeable doer is someone who can appreciate the difference(s) between a caring person (who as a good doer is able to help the child in difficulty) and a therapist who is able, additionally, to help a child take personal responsibilities for his behaviour and then guide the child through to his or her own solutions?

Whether the care is provided by a good doer or a knowledgeable one, the actual delivery of care will not always run smoothly. On admission to a day or residential care setting, and within the context of his or her one-to-one and group interactions, many emotionally disturbed children will seek out ways of presenting to nursing staff the extremely maladapted behaviours which they have learned to use (with some notable successes) in their family, school and neighbourhood environments.

For example, for whatever reasons, one spectrum of maladapted behaviour includes that of being uncooperative or defiant and stubborn to a degree which can be reasonably judged severe enough to interfere with the child's lifestyle and that of others. Nevertheless, if on the one hand individual children can be granted to have varying rights to participate in the prescribing of care in his or her best interests, have they then an equal right to refuse to accept the care which nurses provide? If not, why not? If, however, they do have the right to refuse even some nursing care, how best can that be recognized and appropriate criteria formulated? Furthermore, in making such decisions, to what extent can nurses reasonably make a difference between a child's refusal to accept the care which he or she has helped to decide on and the care which nurses, in exercising their right to implement the Law of Beneficence, have decided he or she must have?

Whether or not any rights to refuse nursing care can be determined and formulated will not really worry many severely disturbed children. Regardless of what nurses [and others] may think, the children present very marked refusals to participate in their physical and psychosocial care. Whenever that happens the problem for nurses is what to do in response to each refusal. Within the realities of their one-to-one and group interactions with children who are not well disposed to meeting people half-way, what strategies do nurses have to make an ethically accepted response?

Nurses are also frequently faced with children who are quite willing to accept the care which they have to offer but non-too-happy to accept that being offered by the other members of the multidisciplinary team, for example medication and individual psychotherapy. In such circumstances nurses are faced with the difficult problem of having to determine whether there can ever be instances whereby a child's refusal to accept non-nursing care can be viewed as a matter of concern, responsibility and action? In such instances, with whom, if anyone, should nurses discuss what their response ought to be?

Yet more issues arise for nurses when it becomes clear that their prescribed care is not having the desired outcome. The reasons may be that the strategy of care being used had not been selected and/or written-up as carefully as it might have, the child may in fact have reacted in a manner which had not been considered very likely, or an unexpected circumstance had arisen (for example, the acute presentation of an infrequent need or problem). The immediate issue is that of identifying the instances when things can be safely left well alone until adequate discussion has taken place, and those that are deemed to require that nurses take some kind of action to spontaneously introduce either a modification to the prescribed care or a new strategy altogether. When such instances arise, whom among the nurses later determines the permanency or otherwise of the action(s) taken?

Nurses will inevitably encounter some instances when a member of the nursing staff, a multi-disciplinary colleague or a parent raises objections to an aspect of the nursing care being delivered. Who, first, has the right to be listened to, although not necessary the right to demand action; and, secondly, who can demand that action be taken to change what nurses are doing?

It is in the hustle and bustle of busy units where the nurses are expected (whether reasonably or not) to go about providing the care they have prescribed that they encounter many problems previously considered unlikely. Such an environment lends itself to questions raised by everyday (though nonetheless difficult) ethical issues. To what extent though might the situation begin to ease for nurses if they viewed the doing of care as not so much the real work of their practise, but as something which was at least in equal partnership with everything else they do?

Judging the effectiveness of care

This stage in the practise of nursing involves comparing a child's behaviour (i.e. by now, his or her responses to nursing care) with that which he or she had presented to staff at the time of admission. Thereafter conclusions have to be reached as to whether the outcome is a favourable or an unfavourable one for the child's present and future well-being.

One of the difficulties of course lies in determining the parameters for favourable and unfavourable behavioural outcomes. Is it, for instance, reasonable to conclude that a child's return to his or her pre-problem lifestyle is an acceptable parameter for a favourable outcome, or can the use of parameters which describe behaviour below or above pre-problem standards ever be justified? Can there ever be, for example, a reasonable argument for stating that a child who had been admitted with a high pre-problem standard of behaviour need not return to that level before being judged ready for the cessation of nursing care? Conversely, is it ever acceptable to stipulate that a child with a low pre-problem standard of behaviour cannot be judged ready for the discontinuation of care until he or she has achieved a higher standard? If a range of new parameters can be considered appropriate for a given child, what might the modified standards be and on whom do decisions rest?

Whatever parameters are arrived at, some outcomes will be considered favourable ones, in which case decisions have to be made as to how best the care can be discontinued.

If, though, the outcome is considered an unfavourable one, then questions need to be asked. For example, have the history, diagnosis and the prescription been written up with an adequate degree of accuracy and clarity? If not, what causes can be identified to help explain any of the shortfalls?

The absence of accuracy and clarity may have been caused by the use of a poorly developed (or over-developed) proforma for a nursing history, by a nurse not in possession of sufficient knowledge, skills and attitude having been given the task of compiling a history, or by a nurse who had not been properly briefed and supervised. If any of these instances (or others akin to them) can be established as the cause(s) then to what degree can any one nurse be held responsible? If, though, the cause lies with the child and family, who perhaps have given insufficient, inaccurate or even misleading information, on whom does the responsibility now rest, and wherein does the ethical response(s) now lie.

An unclear nursing diagnosis could have been formulated because the balance between its objectivity and subjectivity had not been therapeutically achieved. In a case such as this, to what degree might the nurse(s) concerned be in need of counselling on matters related to the appropriate clinical application of objectivity and subjectivity, value judgements, inferences and intuition and personal opinion?

An unfavourable outcome may have arisen as a result of a poorly prescribed nursing care plan and for inconsistent delivery of the plan. In such a circumstance, is it the prescribing nurse or those who have provided the care (or both) who should be held accountable? What though of the child whose care has been poorly prescribed on the basis of, say, misleading information having been deliberately given. Can it ever be considered reasonable to hold the child and family even partly responsible, or must nurses always be held liable to bear the full responsibility?

A considerable ethical issue is presented by the concept of the so-called 'resistent child', who even when provided with the highest standards of nursing care will nevertheless present the behaviour indicative of an unfavourable outcome. In the first place, though, is the concept of a child who will not (or cannot) change a helpful one? Whilst it might seemingly be reasonable to argue that all children are amenable to change (because they are after all growing and developing organisms) most nurses can all too easily bring to mind those children whom they were unable to do anything for. To what extent can nurses ever professionally (and comfortably) conclude that nursing care will never have anything to offer the resistent child, and how are they to deal with their anxieties whenever that conclusion is reached?

An outcome which has been judged unfavourable need not, of course, be viewed negatively. Where a child's response to nursing care has not been as desired, the subsequent review of the history, diagnosis, prescription and delivery of care (against, say, a background of not much data having been initially available) may lead to very helpful additions and modifications to what nurses have until then known about the child and family. In turn this might well lead to therapeutic developments in the nursing care which henceforth is to be provided for the child.

A dilemma for nurses lies, therefore, in determining the differentiation between the criteria that will indicate a need to improve their practise of nursing and that which will indicate that time has been needed for the collation and interpretation of the data necessary for the totality of their care.

But what of the process of the judgement of care itself? If the effectiveness of nursing care is to be judged solely on the interpretation of recorded data about a child's behaviour, then what form should the recording instruments take? Is it sufficient for nurses to rely on data recorded in what might be considered a perfectly adequate Nursing Kardex, or does the importance of evaluating the behaviour of self and the other person justify an argument for nurses having recourse to more specific instruments for the recording of human behaviour? If so, what safeguards might be needed to reduce (or prevent) the tendency for paperwork to dehumanize behaviour.

Even if some form of recorded data is considered necessary, to what extent might it be desirable for nurses to additionally take into account those observations of behaviour which are so subtle as to defy both verbal and written description, but which nevertheless nurses' education, training and experience leads them to conclude are important.

Undoubtedly questions of emotional, social and educational values loom rather large in this final stage in the practise of nursing. In making judgements about the effectiveness or otherwise of their care nurses must inevitably reach conclusions about the behaviour of other people. Therein lie questions about the nature of the parameters for professional conduct, who decides these and what criteria ought they to use?

SOME IMPLICATIONS FOR NURSE EDUCATION AND TRAINING

The profession readily acknowledges that its practitioners (and those in training) ought to be ethics-minded, as they ought to be research-minded.

Paradoxically, one problem for the profession is that the styles with which the practise of nursing is led and managed can be so hierarchical and paternalistic, and quite possibly too influenced by medically based and multi-disciplinary based decisions, as to make the provision of education and training more difficult than it need be. It is probable, then, that the practitioners need to formulate the criteria which will help them identify the circumstances and opportunities which they consider will best promote their education and training in ethical matters. Given the limitations within which this task may have to be undertaken many nurses (acting individually and collectively) will need to be highly motivated and very competent in the practise of assertive skills.

In child psychiatric nursing the required basic content of education and training in ethics, and in the process of decision-making in ethical matters, need not be so dissimilar to that for other areas of nursing as to justify any significant special considerations. The differences in the application of theory and acquired skills which may be implied between the nursing of adults and that of children can usually be adequately attended to through the medium of supervision in the appropriate clinical areas. It is questions about the point at which the supervision of education and training starts and ends and the right to exercise professional accountability and responsibility begins, and who decides on these matters, which are of more immediate importance.

Nurses who work in day and residential units for emotionally disturbed children know only too well the demands and stresses which arise from the constant need to provide a quality of care which can be considered as being in the best interests of each child and family. Strong feelings of inadequacy, frustration, ambivalence and anger are at varying times directed towards self, colleagues and the child. The good nurse willingly accepts experiencing these feelings, agrees that they are uncomfortable and difficult to deal with, and because of this will eagerly seek sources of support. A programme of nurse education and training in ethics must surely be considered inadequate if it has nothing to provide for the support of staff as they encounter the fundamental ethical issues which are part of their everyday practise of nursing. Whatever systems of support is evolved its aims ought to include an examination of the nature of nurses' uncertainties about ethical matters, the identification of personal and collective strengths and from these the establishment of a foundation upon which further levels of expertise can be developed.

The area of ethical issues in the practise of nursing in child psychiatry, like that of many other areas of paediatric nursing, remains one in which there is an urgent need for serious study. Hopefully this book (this chapter in particular for nurses in child psychiatry) will be a key to much needed progress.

ACKNOWLEDGEMENTS

My thanks to Miss L.M. Kitson (Director of Nurse Education) and Mr M. McEwan (Senior Tutor, Psychiatry), both of the Western College of Nursing Midwifery, Greater Glasgow Health Board, for their encouragement and support.

REFERENCES

Hamilton, W.B. (1988) *Nursing in Child, Adolescent and Family Psychiatry: a bibliography with selected annotations.* 7th edn, McEwan Publications, Glasgow (Details from chapter author).

United Kingdom Central Council for Nursing, Midwifery and Health Visiting (1984) *Code of Professional Conduct for the Nurse, Midwife and Health Visitor.* 2nd edn, UKCC, London.

United Kingdom Central Council for Nursing (1986) *Project 2000: a new preparation for practise.* UKCC, London.

United Kingdom Central Council for Nursing (1987a) *Confidentiality. An elaboration of Clause 9 of the second edition of the UKCCs Code of Professional for the Nurse, Midwife and Health Visitor.* UKCC, London.

United Kingdom Central Council for Nursing (1987b) 'Confidentiality'. *Register,* Issue 1, pp 3–4.

6

Ethical issues in the care of the profoundly multiply-handicapped child

PHILIP DARBYSHIRE

HISTORICAL VIEWS OF THE PROFOUNDLY MULTIPLY-HANDICAPPED CHILD

Any discussion of the ethical problems involved in caring for children who are profoundly multiply-handicapped should begin with an examination of their ethical status. Who, or what are they?

Traditionally the profoundly multiply-handicapped child has been viewed as being at the bottom of a very deep barrel. Indeed if it is true that services for mentally handicapped people are the Cinderella services then, to paraphrase the memorable comment of one psychiatric nurse, the profoundly multiply-handicapped child can claim to have been treated as her illegitimate offspring.

How we describe or label someone says a great deal about how we will or should think about them. When the Mental Deficiency Act of 1913 described mentally handicapped people as 'imbeciles', 'morons', 'feeble-minded' or 'moral defectives', this was no value-neutral attempt at classifying people so that appropriate services could be tailored to meet their needs. This was official endorsement of the accepted view that such children were less than human. In one of the most influential textbooks of the day, Treadgold (1937) described profoundly mentally handicapped people thus: 'They have eyes but they see not; ears but they hear not; they have no intelligence and no consciousness of pleasure or pain; in fact their mental state is one of entire negation'.

More recently terminology such as 'high', 'low' and 'medium' grade had a similar effect and the richly abusive language of institutions continues this theme. Profoundly multiply handicapped children have been described as the 'cabbage patch kids' who lived in the 'cot and chair ward' or the 'vegetable patch' (Alaszewski, 1986).

HUMANITY AND PERSONHOOD

This raises the important ethical issue of the humanity or personhood of the profoundly multiply-handicapped child and the direct implications that this question has for the nursing care of these children.

When we consider the severity and extent of the many problems which may affect the profoundly multiply-handicapped child (Table 6.1), the question arises as to whether such a child can really be a human or a person in any sense of the word.

The issue of personhood is a vast and difficult area where even the most expert philosophers are often in deep disagreement and a detailed discussion of this subject is outwith the scope of this chapter. I wish to concentrate, therefore, on one aspect of the issue; that of the characteristics of a person.

In the traditional Judeo–Christian view, all creatures have what Robertson (1975) calls 'a spark of the divine', that is that all human beings are of equal value and have an inherent humanity and personhood. However over the last 15 to 20 years there has been increasing controversy surrounding this question of personhood. If we say that we respect persons so much as an ethical principle, what then is it that we have such respect for?

Table 6.1 One or more of the following features are often found in the profoundly multiply-handicapped child

---

1. Complete absence of speech;
2. Makes no attempt at self help skills, e.g. feeding, dressing;
3. Is doubly incontinent; not toilet trained at all;
4. Has serious sensory deficits, e.g. impaired sight, hearing;
5. Has severe physical handicaps which usually result in a marked degree of immobility;
6. Does not engage in any constructive play with any objects;
7. Seems not to understand any attempt at communication;
8. Apparently lacks recognition of familiar people;
9. Shows little or no reaction to even the most pronounced social stimuli.

Source: Darbyshire, 1986.

Several philosophers, most notably Mary-Anne Warren, Michael Tooley, Joseph Fletcher and Peter Singer have taken the view that to be, or more properly to become, a person you must possess certain qualities or characteristics. Among the most frequently suggested of these are:

1. A person is a subject of non-monetary interests;
2. A person is an entity that possesses rationality;
3. A person is an entity that is capable of action;
4. A person is an entity that possesses self-consciousness.

(Tooley, 1985).

Significantly, many of these characteristics relate to the concept of intelligence. Indeed Fletcher (1972) has seriously suggested that

Any individual of the species *Homo sapiens* who falls below the IQ 40 mark in a standard Stanford–Binet test . . . is questionably a person; below the 20 mark, not a person.

Clearly, using this approach would lead to the conclusion that very few, if any, profoundly multiply-handicapped children could be considered to be persons. The more dramatic implications of such an approach are clear. For example Fletcher sees nothing morally wrong in the killing of such 'non-persons' and Tooley extends this reasoning to allow for infanticide of very young babies, again on the grounds that they are not yet persons. However I do not wish to enter into this area of the dramatic ethical issue since nurses are, unfortunately, rarely intentionally or officially involved in these discussions and decisions.

The question of the personhood and humanity of the profoundly multiply-handicapped child is of crucial importance for nurses. Indeed it seems almost self-evident that in order to provide nursing care in a compassionate and effective way, the nurse must have a clear idea of how he or she perceives the recipient of this care. I will suggest that for nurses, the criteria or characteristics approach to determining personhood is fraught with difficulties.

The first problem is that in isolating sets of characteristics or criteria which are thought to confer membership of the person category, we separate properties from people in a way that is the antithesis of the humanistic and holistic care which nurses are increasingly trying to practise.

Secondly, in attempting to confer personhood by selected

characteristics we create a group of people worthy of our complete respect: persons, and another group or groups who do not fulfil the set criteria and who must by definition be viewed as less than persons and hence be according less respect, or at least a different kind of respect. Yet again, it seems that the mentally handicapped child is born to fail.

Thirdly, it seems that advocates of the characteristics approach have viewed personhood in a philosophical vacuum and have abstracted it out of the context which gives the term so much of its meaning. Perhaps this is why one reviewer of Tooley's book: *Abortion and Infanticide*

> . . . looked in Tooley's index for entries on "Parent", "Mother", "Father", or "Family" and found none.
>
> (Sommers, 1985).

Possibly as a result of this approach, proponents of the characteristics of personhood approach tend to ignore the problem of how such 'non-persons' as the profoundly multiply-handicapped child should be treated (Moskop, 1984). It is difficult to imagine a situation in which nurses could comfortably work within an ethical framework which viewed profoundly multiply-handicapped children as non-persons. For example, I would not like to be the first nurse who tried to argue before a UKCC Disciplinary Committee that her negligence or ill-treatment of a profoundly multiply-handicapped child was not an offence because the child was not a person!

A fourth difficulty with the characteristics approach is in trying to determine the moral significance of the chosen characteristics. Why, for example, should a high IQ score be so worthy of our respect? According to Tooley's criteria Adolph Hitler would be classed as a person, yet many people would have no difficulty in according more respect to the most profoundly handicapped or profoundly multiply-handicapped children.

Finally, despite the insistence of supporters of the characteristics approach that personhood is a state which is gradually achieved, the effect of this approach seems destined to promote the opposite view. Personhood is in danger of being seen as something, like style, that you either do or don't possess. To adopt this position, which sees people as static and non-developing, runs contrary to the value and aims of most nurses working with profoundly multiply-handicapped children.

An essential personal attribute of mental handicap nurses must surely be a sense of optimism that the handicapped child, regardless of the severity of handicap, is capable of making improvements – however undramatic these may seem (Aspin, 1982).

THE ETHICAL STATUS OF THE PROFOUNDLY MULTIPLY-HANDICAPPED CHILD

How then can nurses view the profoundly multiply-handicapped child in such a way as to enhance the nature and effectiveness of the caring relationship which exists between them? Kopelman (1984) argues that:

The notion that we inspect human beings for certain necessary traits, such as sufficient potential for rationality or intelligence, to determine if they are worthy of consideration and care seems improbable when we consider social and family relationships, friendships and affection.

We could more profitably view personhood as a social role rather than as a purely philosophical definition. Babies and young children are conceived within human relationships by parents who are 'morally committed to [its] care on arrival' (Sommers, 1985). Therefore, as Engelhardt (1977) states:

We thus create instead a social sense of person. Children, at least small infants, are persons within the fabric of the social role, "child".

In this context it is often helpful to think of the profoundly multiply-handicapped child as a child first and foremost, albeit one who has very serious handicaps. Ward (1986) adds a further dimension to this social role when he suggests that:

. . . in giving a morally relevant description of a person, we need to mention what she could or might have done, and not just all that she did.

The profoundly multiply-handicapped child therefore has a past as well as a present and, it is to be hoped, a distinct future. This concept is illustrated vividly in one unit where children who have become profoundly multiply-handicapped as a result of progressive neurological disorders, metabolic disorders or accidents have photographs and momentoes from earlier years beside their bed or locker. These are tangible reminders of the child's past as a person which can help nurses to more readily accept their current status as persons despite the extent of their handicaps.

Kopelman (1984) argues that there are three main reasons why profoundly multiply-handicapped children are owed our respect:

First, they share a capacity to feel and their sentience should be respected. Second, . . . how they are treated affects our institutions; thus, it is in our own self-interests to see that they are treated respectfully. Third, beyond the minimal requirements of sentience and self-interest, we share our communities and homes with them; we respect the commitment, benevolent concern or affection that holds families and communities together.

The second of these reasons is especially important for nurses, for if we do not consider these children to be persons then some very real difficulties are created. There are numerous examples in the literature of the poor quality of care that can result when care staff come to accept that the individuals in their care are somehow less than persons or less than human (Beardshaw, 1981; Martin and Evans, 1984).

Institutional care was often accused of de-humanizing or de-personalizing people, and with good reason. The acceptance of the view that profoundly multiply-handicapped children are less than persons can give rise to extremely negative patterns of nursing care, characterized by ways of thinking exemplified in the 'ten institutional why's':

1. Why talk to them – they can't hear;
2. Why listen to them – they can't tell us anything;
3. Why ask them – they can't choose;
4. Why teach them – they can't learn;
5. Why show them – they can't see;
6. Why give them good food – they can't taste any difference;
7. Why change them – they'll only wet and soil again;
8. Why give them toys – they can't play;
9. Why take them out – they don't notice anything;
10. Why bother . . .?

Apart from the more obvious effects of such negative views of profoundly multiply-handicapped children on the care of the child, there is a less often discussed but equally destructive effect upon nurses themselves. Working with profoundly multiply-handicapped children over a long period of time is extremely demanding. For nurses to maintain a high level of commitment, enthusiasm and humanity is not easy. Sadly many staff in such areas become disillusioned, defeatist and cynical (Firth *et al*, 1987). Some burn-out even before they have caught fire.

To help combat these occupational hazards it would help if nurses working with profoundly multiply-handicapped children were to participate in values clarification exercises to discuss and clarify their thoughts regarding the moral and ethical issues which are relevant to their work (Colletta, 1978). Such exercises are sorely needed if nurses are to develop a coherent philosophy which will underpin the care given in the ward or unit. All too often such issues are simply ignored or discussion is actively discouraged. For example, a student nurse on her first day in a unit for profoundly multiply-handicapped children asked the routine question 'Where is the resuscitation equipment?'. The Staff Nurse looked at her in disbelief and replied, 'You won't need that here'. The point here is not the rights and wrongs of resuscitation for these children but the way in which ethical issues are decided on an *ad hoc* basis, in Masonic secrecy and with seemingly no recognition that these are issues worthy of discussion.

I suggest that profoundly multiply-handicapped children should be seen as not only deserving of our care, based upon the moral principles of beneficence, justice, and respect for persons, but as children who have an extraordinary need to be valued for what they are and for what they may yet become. We need to see these children not as permanently lacking in essential attributes, but as being primarily children with a capacity for development, however limited that may be. For nurses to develop positive attitudes towards the care of the profoundly multiply-handicapped child, ethical thinking and discussion is essential. Indeed, it could be claimed that the teaching of ethics provides the firmest ground for the attainment of high nursing standards or quality of care. In this section I have tried to trace some historical threads in ethical thinking and the implications that this has for the profoundly multiply-handicapped child, and to counter some of the argumets put forward by those who see personhood as being characterized by a set of abilities. My basic proposition is in fact very simple; that nurses must regard profoundly multiply-handicapped children not simply as persons but as exceptional persons, because ultimately there is no other feasible alternative for nurses or nursing.

Mary Warnock has said that:

The question must ultimately be, what kind of society can we praise and admire: In what kind of society can we live with our conscience clear.

(cited by Steinbock, 1985).

I do not believe that nurses could take pride in their care of profoundly multiply-handicapped children in an environment where such children were seen as *persona non grata*.

ETHICAL PRINCIPLES: CAN THEY HELP?

There is no doubt that working with profoundly multiply-handicapped children can be extremely demanding both physically and emotionally, and it is not difficult to see how the consideration of ethical issues can seem to be the least of nurses' problems. In wards or units for profoundly multiply-handicapped children nurses are frequently in the position of rushing to get the work done, either to get children up and dressed in time for breakfast, or to get breakfast over in time for school, or to get children to bed before night staff come on duty. The list of deadlines confronting staff provides a relentless focus on the speedy completion of physical tasks and with this comes an emphasis on the skills, not of thoughtful, intelligent and considerate care, but of speed and the ability to master the ward routine. In the midst of this headlong rush to get the work done suggestions that nurses stop for a while and allow time to identify and discuss ethical issues is likely to be met with less than wild enthusiasm. However I suggest that such thought given to the ethical issues which face all nurses caring for profoundly multiply-handicapped children would pay real dividends for both staff and children.

A real difficulty for nurses in this situation is in actually identifying ethical issues and problems. We are all familiar with the ethical and moral dilemmas which tend to attract the headlines and attention, for example, should profoundly multiply-handicapped babies be 'allowed to die' in certain circumstances or should severely mentally handicapped young women be sterilized to prevent their having children, or should profoundly multiply-handicapped children be allowed to have major surgery in order to prolong their lives. For nurses, however, there are many ethical issues which face them in their daily work which are of equal importance, for how they are dealt with affects not only the nurse but in very definite ways affects the quality of life of the profoundly multiply-handicapped children in their care.

Nurses can recognize ethical issues when they begin to ask the 'What should be done?', 'What ought I to do?', 'What is best for ...?', 'Is it right to ...', 'Do I have the right to ...?', 'Will this benefit or harm ...?', 'Who is responsible for ...?' and other questions which involve normative or value statements. These issues are clearly different from other aspects of care such as the technical or even the legal aspects. For example, it is possible for a nurse to perform the passing of a naso–gastric tube and administer a tube-feed in a faultlessly technical way, however if the nurse did not ask the person's permission, or did not explain exactly what was happening, or was not truthful about the purpose of the tube, or if the tube was being passed into the stomach of a comatose person who had expressly requested that no lift-sustaining measures such as this be taken when he or she had written a 'living will', then the nurses ethical competence is less certain.

When nurses begin to identify the many ethical aspects of their work they are still faced with the problem of how to nurse profoundly multiply-handicapped children in ways which are ethically acceptable. Despite the many differences of opinion which exist between ethicists and philosophers, there are some ethical principles which are almost universally accepted and which can help nurses to make the best decisions when faced with the dilemmas that caring for profoundly multiply-handicapped children can pose.

These are: respect for persons and their autonomy, justice and equal and fair treatment, honesty and truthfulness, beneficence; the principle of doing good not harm and the duty of care to fellow beings, non-maleficence; the principle of doing no harm. At first glance, such principles seem simple, almost too simple, after all there can be few nurses who disagree with the idea of doing good for people as opposed to harming them. However, these principles can become very complex especially when principles seem to be competing against each other and choices have to be made.

Respect for persons and their autonomy

The previous discussion of the personhood of profoundly multiply-handicapped children was intended to establish that such children are worthy of our respect as persons. But we are confronted with an equally difficult problem when we try to establish their autonomy. Indeed for the profoundly multiply handicapped child, who may be unable to communicate by speech or gesture and who may be virtually immobile due to severe physical handicaps, it seems that his or her autonomy and decision-making capacity are non-existent. As Gillon (1986) notes 'The crucial question then arises, how much autonomy does a person need to have for his autonomy to require respect?'. In such cases surely the nurse is justified in adopting a paternalistic approach whereby he or she will make all of the decisions about the child's daily life but with their best interests at heart. He or she will look after them for their own good. As is so often the case when it appears that ethical principles are in conflict, in this case, autonomy and beneficence and the duty to care, the nurse is faced with an ethical choice about his or her possible nursing actions.

The problem of the impaired autonomy of profoundly multiply-handicapped children must be resolved by accepting the fact that in most cases the nurse's duty to care and the child's best interests will be the overriding considerations. However, it is important that in accepting this position that the nurse also accepts that this is not the same as saying that profoundly multiply-handicapped children have no autonomy. They still have very definite rights; to explanations geared to their level of understanding however impaired this may be, to have preferences sought and respected whenever possible and to have their body privacy and dignity respected. Indeed it could be argued that when a child's autonomy is severely impaired the nurse has an increased responsibility to ensure that their personhood and essential humanity is respected. This is an awesome challenge for any nurse, to try to put himself or herself in the position of the profoundly multiply-handicapped child through his or her skills in human relationships and in a sense be the child's autonomy (see Case 1 at the end of this chapter).

If autonomy is accepted as a valuable ethical principle then nurses will want to consider ways in which they might increase the autonomy of the profoundly multiply-handicapped child. This may not be as impossible as it may first appear but it is important that any plans to achieve this are realistic. It is not realistic to expect a profoundly multiply-handicapped child to be able to make major decisions about every aspect of their lives, but small and significant steps can be made. Since a large part of the day in wards or units for profoundly multiply-handicapped children will be taken up by physical care work such as bathing, feeding, dressing and changing this could provide a focus for any interventions aimed at giving the children an increased sense of autonomy. An essential element of this autonomy is that the child is given a choice and subsequently thinks and decides freely what choice they will make. Through this process the child learns that they matter and that their decisions, however small, make a difference in their lives. Profoundly multiply-handicapped children can be offered such small choices regardless of the severity of their handicaps. Experienced nurses who work with profoundly multiply-handicapped children often say that they are all different, all individuals, that they all have their own unique personalities, their own likes and dislikes. Recognition of this fact is the basis for encouraging the child to learn to make choices for themselves.

The important thing is to encourage the choice and be prepared to accept the child's indication of preference wherever possible. For example the child could be offered the choice of two dresses or shirts to wear and may be able to indicate or learn how to indicate their preference. Similarly at mealtimes any food preferences which the child has could be encouraged and respected although again if the child wishes to eat only ice-cream then the principle of beneficence and paternalism in the child's best interests would doubtless override their wishes! This discussion of autonomy and encouraging choices in profoundly multiply-handicapped children may seem very academic and unimportant but it is an issue which has major implications for the way that nurses work with such children. Not only are such children's personhood and humanity enhanced when nurses begin to consider that they have a right to be asked and consulted about the seemingly trivial things in life which we take so much for granted (who chooses what you will wear each morning, or what you will have for lunch?), but there is the possibility of a knock-on effect which will touch other areas of the child's total care. If nurses see that a child is able to learn to express a preference in however limited a fashion, they will then begin to think of other things that they may be capable of learning or of other ways in which this sense of being may be channelled.

There are other aspects of the principles of respect for persons which have a direct bearing on the work of nurses who care for profoundly multiply-handicapped children. These are issues related to privacy, respect for human dignity and integrity, individualization and the commitment of nursing to treat children as individuals. The idea that, as nurses, we treat each patient as an individual is put forward so often without any thought as to its myriad implications that we are in danger of rendering the concept meaningless. Yet these concepts which at first glance seem to be more related to ordinary politeness are in fact important ethical issues related to the child's personhood and autonomy. It is not merely impolite to be changing a profoundly multiply-handicapped child while talking to a colleague and ignoring the child, or to pick up the child without trying to tell them that you are about to do so and what you are about to do with them, it is also ethically poor nursing practise.

Beneficence and nonmaleficence

This often seems to be the most obvious and uncontentious of all ethical principles, after all what reasonable nurse could possibly disagree with the idea that we should try to do that which will benefit the child and refrain from any actions that will cause the child harm? This is a principle that has been enshrined in many of nursing's ethical codes, for example the *Code of Professional Conduct for the Nurse, Midwife and Health Visitor* issued by the UKCC says that the nurse shall:

Act always in such a way as to promote and safeguard the well-being and interests of patients/clients

and that they shall:

Ensure that no action or omission on his/her part or within his/her sphere of influence is detrimental to the condition or safety of patients/clients.

However these principles are in reality fraught with difficulty as they often seem to be in conflict with each other and clear cut examples of what is good for and what is bad for the child are rare. The nurse's view of doing good for the profoundly multiply-handicapped child might be that he or she should do everything for them as they are so extensively handicapped, but this raises the question of whether he or she is in a sense harming the child by limiting their autonomy and their right to the level of independence they may be capable of achieving, however minimal this might be.

It is also difficult to decide whether in practice these two principles have equal importance, or in what circumstances one principle should override the other. For example, a nurse might decide that a profoundly multiply-handicapped child is so physically fragile that they should not be taken out of their bed for play sessions as the activities could cause them harm despite the benefits that are claimed for the play.

Another problem relates to the previous discussion of autonomy and the principle of respecting a child's wishes. There may be occasions when unpleasant or even painful procedures may be performed on the profoundly multiply-handicapped child, who shows signs of pain and distress at these interventions. This raises the question of whether it is acceptable to inflict this distress in the short-term as the long-term benefits may be thought to outweigh this (see Case 2 at the end of this chapter).

The principles of beneficence and nonmaleficence raise many other questions which are perhaps more difficult to answer, for example should we consider only the child or do questions of good and harm involve not only the child but the family and indeed the community and society itself?

Justice

The principle of justice, incorporating the ideals of fairness, equality and non-discrimination, tends to be discussed in relation to larger issues such as the allocation of resources. Discussions of this subject are an almost constant feature in newspaper articles and TV documentaries. Should the health services resources be spent on preventative care or on acute hospitals? Should transplant surgery programmes be allocated finance in preference to services for elderly people or mentally handicapped people? These, and similar grand questions, may make us feel that the principle of justice has little relevance for everyday nursing practise with profoundly multiply-handicapped children, but this is not the case. Nurses are faced with questions related to justice and fairness every time that they decide on their nursing priorities and how they will allocate their time. Nurses' time is after all an extremely valuable resource and it should be valued enough for its use to be carefully considered. Nurses are inevitably faced with decisions about how best to deploy available staff but it is often assumed that this is purely a ward management decision when in fact it is often a decision which has a strong ethical component (see Case 3 at the end of this chapter).

ARE NURSES FREE TO TAKE ETHICAL DECISIONS?

One important question which must be faced when discussing how nurses can nurse ethically is, are nurses in the position of being able to be ethical? How much autonomy do nurses themselves have when it comes to making their ethical decisions? Can they decide on ethical courses of nursing action independently or are there constraints which prevent them from doing so or severely modify their decisions?

These questions are vitally important as they affect every nurse's ethical behaviour, unfortunately the answers to the questions which are raised are much less clear. Two interesting papers recently argued these issues of nurses' autonomy and freedom to make ethical decisions. Yarling and McElmurray (1986) argued that 'nurses are often not free to be moral' and that they were restrained and inhibited by the bureaucratic nature of the hospital, by the greater power and authority of doctors and senior nurses and by their traditional roles as recipients of orders rather than as decision-makers in their own right. They also argue that what nurses are taught officially during their training is cancelled out by the powerful influence of the practices which occur in the wards of the hospital to which they must ultimately fit in, or as they put it, 'Professional nurses are conceived in moral contradiction and born in compromise'. These authors suggest that the answers to this problem is that nursing must somehow:

. . . acquire sufficient power within the hospital, relative to medicine and administration to create a balance of power in the control of the practice or it must terminate its employee status with the hospital, move outside the hospital, and serve hospital patients from the vantage point of some new nursing-controlled organisation.

(Yarling and McElmurray, 1986).

In contrast to this radical proposal (Bishop and Scudder, 1987) suggest that a more reforming solution is both possible and desirable. They argue that Yarling and McElmurray (1986) ignore the fact that on numerous occasions throughout the day nurses do nurse ethically despite the many demands and constraints placed upon them. They cite the work of Benner in emphasizing that this is an essential aspect of professional competence, the

coping with staff shortages [by] maintaining a caring attitude towards patients even in the absence of close and frequent contact.

They also suggest that hospitals are perhaps too easy to cast into the role of the 'bad guy' and claim that,

Institutions afford security, stable financial support, facilities, and resources to their members. If one receives these benefits, then one usually pays a price – often loss of some individual freedom.

Bishop and Scudder (1987) also argue that demands for excessive autonomy can lead to increasing conflict within groups of staff and that nurses occupy a unique in-between position in respect of the patient, the medical staff and the hospital which could be used to promote more cooperative and mutually acceptable ethical decisions.

CONCLUSIONS AND SUGGESTIONS

In this chapter I have tried to establish an ethical basis for the nursing care of the profoundly multiply-handicapped child. This basis is the humanity and personhood of the child which is an inherent aspect of the social role of being a child and is not determined by characteristics such as intelligence or abilities. Fundamental ethical principles were outlined and ways in which these might help nurses to think ethically about the care that they give to profoundly multiply-handicapped children were discussed. The difficulties which can arise when trying to apply moral principles were also discussed.

If all of these issues seem difficult it is because they are difficult. Nobody has ever suggested that nursing well was easy. But they are concepts which nurses can become more familiar with and more expert at discussing and using, providing of course that they have been recognized as being important and worthy of the nurse's consideration.

The quality of nursing care that profoundly multiply-handicapped children receive is dependent upon many factors, of which the ethical self-awareness of their nurses is one of the most pivotal. When nurses evaluate the care of a profoundly multiply-handicapped child in terms of how their development has been encouraged, how individualized their care has been, how they have been helped to integrate with the community at large, how they have been involved in pleasurable experiences, how they have been helped to stay in the best possible physical and nutritional condition, how they have been communicated with and had their attempts at communication attended to and how they have been generally loved and cared for; for good nursing is an emotional as well as a practical activity, then they are evaluating what Bishop and Scudder (1987) call 'the moral sense of nursing'. Children at their most vulnerable and dependent have every right to expect this of us.

CASE 1

Mary is a four-year-old child who has been profoundly multiply-handicapped since birth as a result of perinatal trauma. She is fed a liquidized or soft diet which she takes very slowly, and sometimes reluctantly, from a spoon. Student nurse Wilson was giving Mary her lunch when staff nurse Smith came up to her and began to complain about how long she was taking to feed her. She told her that there were more children in the ward than just Mary and that as a result of her taking so long they were 'starving'. Mary was having her liquidized main course and staff nurse Smith told student nurse Wilson to 'just mix the pudding in with it' as this would help her to finish more quickly and let the domestic staff get the meal trolley ready in time for its return to the hospital kitchen. Student nurse Wilson was unhappy about this and told staff nurse Smith that she did not think it was right to offer Mary something to eat that she herself found to be quite revolting. Staff nurse Smith said that normally she would agree but that Mary was so severely handicapped that it was unlikely that she was capable of tasting food in the normal sense of the word so this was a foolish argument, and that, in any case, the needs of the rest of the children took precedence over those of one child.

CASE 2

Sally is eight years old and has become profoundly multiply-handicapped as a result of a rare metabolic disease which is becoming progressively worse. The staff were worried that she was becoming increasingly immobile and was beginning to develop positional deformities of her hips and spine as a result of this. The physiotherapists designed a special lying-frame for Sally made from wood covered in soft foam which was designed to place Sally in an anatomically good position when she was lying down. In this way it was hoped that her positional deformities would be prevented or at least minimized or delayed. However, Sally seemed to hate lying in this frame and would grimace and make a very quiet crying sound when put in it. This was very unusual for Sally as the nurses considered that she was virtually incapable of making any recognizable display of either pleasure or distress. They decided that this was significant and that they would observe Sally closely. Over the next week or two they did this and Sally continued to seem distressed when placed in the frame. One day when staff nurse White was on duty Sally had seemed to be more distressed than usual. She told another member of staff that she had had enough of 'seeing Sally suffer like this' and asked for help to take her out of the frame and lie her on top of the bed. When this was done Sally immediately seemed less distressed. Later that afternoon the physiotherapist visited and immediately asked why Sally was not in her frame. Staff nurse White explained about Sally's 'distress' but the physiotherapist said that this was normal for the child to protest initially but that 'they always get used to it in time' and insisted that staff nurse White put Sally back in the frame. Staff nurse White refused, saying that she had a responsibility to protect Sally from harm and distress and to respect her wishes wherever possible and that clearly she did not wish to lie in the frame. She also said that as Sally's condition was progressive and as she was not expected to live for more than perhaps a year or two, that it was foolish to subject her to discomfort and distress for some long-term gains that she may never live to benefit from. The physiotherapist left, threatening to report staff nurse Smith to the ward sister and to Sally's consultant.

CASE 3

Staff nurse Jones had worked in the unit for profoundly multiply-handicapped children for several years and had developed a strong bond of affection with all of the children, but especially with Robert who had lived in the unit for almost all of his seven years. However, his parents had had to move home to work in another part of the country and Robert was to move to a unit near their new home. Staff nurse Jones was sad that Robert was leaving but his parents had said how good the new unit seemed to be so that was reassuring. Staff nurse Jones had arranged with Robert's parents and the ward sister that as a special treat on his last day in the unit, she would take Robert to the zoo, which he really loved, and then back to the unit for a special leaving party. Nurse Jones had put a great deal of her own time and effort into this trip and to the party. She had told Robert all about it and she knew that he was excited and looking forward to it. On the morning of Robert's last day there was a 'phone call for nurse Jones from the nursing administration office telling her that because of a shortage of staff on the busy surgical ward she would have to go there for the day to help out. She explained to the nursing officer about Robert's last day, the trip and the party, but the nursing officer said that she was the only available person who could be sent and that if it wasn't an urgent situation she would not be asked. Nurse Jones argued that she had a strong obligation to keep her promises to Robert and not to disappoint him and that he would be unlikely to understand why the zoo trip would have to be cancelled or why she would not be there at the party to say goodbye. The nursing officer began to lose patience with nurse Jones and reminded her of her obligations to the hospital as a whole, who employed her and paid her salary and also emphasized that in the surgical ward where she was needed, the children there had much more 'serious need of her nursing skills' than would a child for a trip or a party. She told nurse Jones that she should consider whether it is wise to become so over-involved with the children, told her to report to the surgical ward in ten minutes then put down the phone.

DISCUSSION POINTS FOR CASES 1–3

1. What are the ethical principles at issue in each of these cases?
2. Where do these principles seem to come into conflict?
3. Each of the situations in these cases has ultimately ended in conflict and some acrimony. Is this an inevitable feature of ethical disagreements? If it is not, how could a more reasoned and constructive outcome been engineered?
4. What course of action could or should student nurse Wilson, staff nurse White and staff nurse Jones follow in each of the above cases and why?

REFERENCES

Alaszewski, A. (1986) *Institutional Care and the Mentally Handicapped: The mental handicap hospital.* Croom Helm, London.

118 Ethics in paediatric nursing

Aspin, D.N. (1982) Towards a concept of human being as a basis for a philosophy of special education. *Education Review*, **34** (2), 113–23.

Beardshaw, V. (1981) *Conscientious Objectors at Work: Mental hospital nurses – a case study*. Social Audit, London.

Bishop, A.H. and Sudder, J.R. Jnr. (1987) Nursing ethics in an age of controversy. *Adv. Nurs. Sci.*, **9** (3), 34–43.

Colletta, S.S. (1978) Values clarification in nursing: Why? *Amer. J. Nurs.*, Dec, 2057–63.

Darbyshire, P. (1986) Physical aspects of care of the profoundly multiply handicapped. In E. Shanley (ed.), *Mental Handicap: a handbook of care*. Churchill Livingstone, Edinburgh.

Engelhardt Jnr, H.T. (1977) Some persons are humans, some humans are persons, and the world is what we make it. In S.F. Spicker and H.T. Engelhardt Jnr (eds), *Philosophical Medical Ethics: its nature and significance*. D. Reidel Pub. Co., Dordrecht.

Firth, H., McKeown, P., McIntee, J. and Britton, P. (1987) Professional depression, 'burnout' and personality in longstay nursing. *Int. J. Nurs. Stud.*, **24** (3), 227–37.

Fletcher, J. (1972) *Indicators of Humanhood: A tentative profile of man*. Hastings Centre Report, **2** (1), 1–4.

Kopelman, L. (1984) Respect and the retarded: issues of valuing and labelling. In L. Kopelman and J.C. Moskop (eds), *Ethics and Mental Retardation*. D. Reidel/Kluwer, Dordrecht.

Martin, J.P. and Evans, D. (1984) *Hospitals in Trouble*. Basil Blackwell, Oxford.

Moskop, J.C. (1984) Responsibility for the retarded: two theoretical views. In L. Kopelman and J.C. Moskop (eds), *Ethics and Mental Retardation*. D. Reidel/Kluwer, Dordrecht.

Robertson (1975) Involuntary euthanasia of defective newborns: a legal analysis. *Stanford Law Review*, **27**, 213–69.

Sommers, C.H. (1985) *Reviews: Tooley's immodest proposal*. Hastings Center Report, June, 39–42.

Steinbock, B. (1985) Infanticide. In R.S. Laura and A.F. Ashman (eds), *Moral Issues in Mental Retardation*. Croom Helm, London.

Tooley, M. (1985) *Abortion and Infanticide*. Clarendon Press/Oxford University Press, Oxford.

Treadgold, A. (1937) *A Textbook of Mental Deficiency*. Williams and Wilkins, Baltimore.

Ward, K. (1986) Persons, kinds and capacities. In P. Byrne (ed.), *Rights and Wrongs in Medicine: King's College Studies 1985–6*. King Edward's Hospital Fund for London/Oxford University Press, London.

Yarling, R.R. and McElmurray, B.J. (1986) The moral foundation of nursing. *Adv. Nurs. Sci.*, **8** (2), 63–73.

7

Ethical considerations in paediatric nursing research

GOSIA M. BRYKCZYŃSKA

It is hard to be overly concerned about the ethics of health-care research, in spite of several nurses recently questioning the extent of the swing of the ethical awareness pendulum (Robb, 1983; Noble, 1985; Melia, 1986). Ethical concerns stemming from the nature of current research are so numerous that all researchers should be obliged to analyse the implications of their work and, short of ethical considerations paralysing research, no moral concern should ever be too great an exaggeration. In the context of nursing, the process of research carries the additional moral obligation of maintaining a covenant relationship with the patient, which is integral to the art of nursing while supporting the promise to care for the patient by looking at the nature and quality of the nursing care.

The nurse undertaking research is trying to improve and advance the quality of nursing care by examining a facet of nursing in a dispassionate and scientific fashion. This can lead, however, to a conflict of professional interests, since the nurse is also expected to be empathetic with the patient. This problem can be overcome to some extent by a re-evaluation of the very concepts of scientific research, such that participant observation research, case review studies and action research all become acceptable forms of nursing research. Not only does such qualitative research confront some of the ethical problems inherent in other research methods more directly, but often this type of research is more appropriate for studying social sciences, especially with a vulnerable population such as patients or children.

Most advances in medicine and nursing have come as a result of intense and prolonged research – often spanning many years. In the field of paediatrics, innovations in practice have come as a result of research work with children, and therefore the single most important concept in the ethical debate concerning research with human subjects is left open for criticism – namely the idea of voluntariness (Fowler, 1987). It is always important that participants of research volunteer, that is, freely agree to participate in the research; however, the issue becomes quite complicated when the human subject is a child, an emotionally unstable adult, or an elderly insane individual (Douglas *et al*, 1986; Culver *et al*, 1980; Erickson, 1987; Shaw, 1973; Silva and Sorrell, 1984).

A child must prove that he or she is aware of the concept of voluntariness and of his or her own free will wishes to participate; and all this on the basis of informed consent. This is, of course, a tall order for adults, let alone a child! (Silva and Sorrell, 1984; Roth *et al*, 1977; Carney, 1987; Karani, 1986). Social psychologists and child developmentalists have looked into the nature of children's cognitive and moral development – most notable amongst these are Jean Piaget and Lawrence Kohlberg, whose work on moral development beautifully illustrates the sequential nature of that development. Kohlberg's work is still being developed and, in the nature of a founding theory, has inconsistencies and irregularities; some of these points he has developed since his first theory was launched, and some have been elaborated by others. Nurses have found Kohlberg's work useful in explaining moral development, e.g. Mahon and Fowler, and especially paediatric nurses and professionals involved in work with children have found the concepts beneficial in approaching a more holistic theory of child development, that is, integrating moral development with social, cognitive and psychological development.

If we assume, therefore, that some form of sequential moral development is operating in the developing child then we can ask the question, at what stage in that moral development is a child ready to volunteer to participate in a research project? Volunteering is, however, not only a moral attribute, it also entails a specific level of cognitive development and social awareness. Fowler explains voluntariness as an alliance of informedness, consent and autonomy – such that in Kantian terms 'truly free choices are examined ones that emanate from one's reason' (Fowler, 1987). With such a definition of volunteering it is hard to see a child below the age of six or seven truly being able to volunteer, and yet children ought to be asked if they want to participate, and even pre-school children are asked if they wish to join a research study. Non-invasive child development studies pose little personal threat to the integrity of pre-school children, e.g. studying children's perceptions of illness, body-parts, health (Eiser, 1983). One such type of research may involve children making illustrations for the researcher. The children under-stand that their drawings are for 'teacher' or 'nurse' and as willingly as they ever do (some children never seem keen to part with their masterpieces), they hand them over to the teacher, nurse or resear-cher who then analyses them for research purposes. This type of developmental work poses few problems and it is heartening to know that child-care workers and paediatric nurse-researchers are increasingly directly asking the children for permission to use children's work in studies; they ask for the children to volunteer in the studies and they listen carefully to youngsters' concerns. They do not only approach parents as has been the traditional custom.

Issues become less clear when the nature of the study is invasive or potentially invasive, even if it carries with it less than minimal risks. It is as well to remember here that the very concept of risk is not uniform either and there is much confusion between lawyers, professionals, patients and the lay public over the definition of reasonable risk-taking (Bracken, 1987). Invasiveness is not only a concept of physiological invasiveness; children sharing ideas about life at home, for the benefit of a researcher, can become just as upset at the insistent questions of researchers, as children having blood samples taken, even if the adults are conducting research which is designed to help the children in the long run. Both events may be seen as an invasion of the child's private world. Given that children have a different perception of the future and, depending on their level of cognitive development, may have limited understanding of time, it should be recognized that agreeing to participate in studies now may not mean that the child is prepared to be in the study tomorrow. It was because of some of these concerns over the developmental status of the child that the post-War codes of experimental medicine and research discouraged the use of children in research – that is, specifically non-therapeutic research.

With the emergence of medicine as a serious scientific discipline 'the birth of the clinic' also heralded a new approach to therapy. With the introduction of novel treatments and experimental medicine, medical research started to follow a scientific approach. The early pioneers of experimental medicine were often Renaissance men of eclectic tastes, and self-motivated; often inflicting possible harm on themselves in order to prove the efficacy of a vaccine or treatment. Such questionable heroism as that of the Scandinavian Dr Daniellson who innoculated himself with the mycobacterium *Leprae* in order to prove the efficacy of his treatment against Hansen's disease was not unusual (Feeny, 1964). This tradition of starting with oneself as research subject (auto-experimentation) is certainly not new and is traditionally followed by the custom of initially trying out one's new discovery on one's wife, children, neighbours and colleagues. The extent to which these people were asked for, and subsequently gave, their consent varied enormously, but the ethical principle underlying the approach was, for the most part, one of unhesitating beneficence and largesse – if somewhat misguided. The greatest flaw in such an approach was the assumption that 'others would automatically do that which I would do, especially those close to me. They would think as I do and wish to behave as I do'. Altruism, however, is a characteristic of moral development that is not readily transferable from one individual to another, although ethical consciousness-raising concerning some matters can increase the manifestations of latent altruism, e.g. one can be encouraged to donate organ parts to a medical school upon death, or to carry a kidney donor card in case of death in the event of a road traffic accident.

After this awkward honeymoon with *ad hoc* research subjects, physicians started to look directly at patients as potential research subjects, and started to institute novel treatment regimes as and when they felt appropriate, with very little regard to what today would be considered research techniques. This approach to the advancement of medical scientific knowledge is typified by the work of Dr Semmelweiss with post-partum mothers (Clendening, 1942). The physician saw it as his or her perogative to administer, alter or introduce whatever treatment seemed appropriate, regardless of its proven efficacy. The concept of initial trials or pilot studies was not yet popular among the medico-scientific community. So long as the physician had a curative end in mind this approach was at least in keeping with the general paternalistic approach to patients which was prevalent at the time. Problems of a serious ethical nature started to emerge however, when patients were catagorized into arbitrary groups by the physicians-cum-researchers, so that any kind of research or experimental medicine was considered 'fair game' in certain populations because of predefined external characteristics of the research population. Heading such a list of research 'conscripted volunteers' must be the legions of prisoners and army recruits (Hodges and Bean, 1967). The vaccination trials for yellow fever and dengue fever were carried out on army recruits by the US Army medical corps in the best of faith – but it seems of questionable ethics today; however science now owes much to the work of those pioneering giants of medicine and unsung heroes of voluntariness.

Sadly, even when it was proven that a particular intervention saved lives and reduced morbidity, it was not always introduced immediately into the general population. British sailors faired well on lime juice with reduced incidence of scurvy compared with American sailors of the same period who were not introduced to the novel dietary regime, even though they knew enough about the diet to name the British sailor a 'limey'. From using army volunteers for medical research to the use of 'volunteers' from institutions was only a matter of time. Children from institutions for the mentally handicapped were used for various research projects, the most notorious such piece of research being conducted at Willowbrook State School, where mentally handicapped youngsters were subjected to live hepatitis virus in order to determine the efficacy of the new hepatitis vaccine, then being developed. This occurred in the early 1960s, but 20 years prior to this a far greater threat to medical and nursing research emerged in the form of medical non-therapeutic experiments on healthy and sick subjects alike during the reign of the Third Reich. The Nazi philosophy at the time in Germany and on occupied territories precluded any notion of consent to research and experiments were conducted on human subjects for a wide variety of scientific projects – one of the least recognized being the scientific basis for the food rations given to the Jewish occupants of the Warsaw Ghetto. This was calculated to starve out the population within 18 months.

The experiments were conducted on a captive population of prisoners in concentration camps or jails. From the atrocities of this period arose the impetus for drawing up an international set of rules governing research with human subjects, and in 1949 the Nuremberg code was proclaimed. As the military tribunals sat in disbelief listening to and witnessing the horrors that the research subjects recounted it became clear that guidelines would be needed to govern the behaviour of physician-researchers, indeed of all researchers working with human subjects. Thus the first attempt at stating what perhaps should have been obvious (but only too patently proved otherwise), was drafted with the Nazi regime atrocities in mind and the first point in that declaration sets out the inviolatable prerequisition for any research using human subjects – that subjects must give their free consent to participation in the study. Since the Nuremberg Declaration several other codes have been drawn up by the international medical and research community; on average an update of the code or a modification has been written every ten years, the most relevant to physicians being the Helsinki Code of 1964. Now with high technology pushing the frontiers of medicine further and further back on each side of the life cycle – and a threat is being posed to the integrity of both the immature and post-mature human individual – a new flurry of international activity can be sensed as research workers, ethicists, and health-care workers begin to question anew the ethics of research on embryos, experimental procedures on fetuses, research on very early premature infants, experiments with fetal tissue, subjecting the elderly frail to technological insults, and so on.

The positive explosion of centres for bio-ethics (almost every country in Europe, North America and Australasia has such a centre), the expansion of departments of moral philosophy and bio-ethics, the institution of new post-graduate programs in medical ethics, and the birth of new journals concerned with ethical issues in health-care, are all reflective of the growing awareness of ethical issues in medicine and the health-care professions. This awareness has now resulted in yet more pressure being exerted on individuals engaged in health-care research so that their work follows the international codes of medical and research practice. Unfortunately, many countries see the codes purely as recommendations, and adherence to these recommendations can be very arbitrary. The recent work of Dutch nurses with survivors of torture can be seen as a bleak reminder that torture still exists, and that it often exists with the consent and co-operation of health-care workers (Tornbjerg and Jacobsen, 1986), in spite of international codes of medical conduct condemning such activities.

Pressures may be put on researchers to adhere to certain recommendations, e.g. all research involving human subjects should be submitted to an ethics committee and professional groups should ensure that no research is published without having first been cleared by an ethics committee. What is still not clear is the nature and functional composition of ethics committees. These measures also do not address the problem of research conducted by researchers outside the domain of medical science, e.g. conducted by physiologists, who can be governed by a different professional group than health-care workers (Rothrock, 1985; Pollock and Tilley, 1987; Shelp and Frost, 1980; Robinson, 1987). These people, if unscrupulous and ethically immature, could work in an unethical fashion but still be beyond the control of health-care professionals or even the law, since the nature of their work tends to be in advance of the law, as in the cases of research into trans-species organ transplantation, fetal tissue transplants and embryo research. Of course sanctions imposed on rights to publish can affect all researchers, but funding contingent on ethicacy of a research project can be less of a problem if the research is privately funded. Even when the law does step in, in the form of formal legislative enquiries and recommendations concerning the nature and method of research, as in the instance of research work into infertility and *in vitro* fertilization with the establishment of the Warnock Committee and its subsequent Report to the public, the recommendations carry little weight. The recommendations of the Warnock Report quickly lost authority as the experimental nature of the procedures investigated increasingly became medical routine, displacing yesterdays ethical problems with a host of new ones.

Various solutions have been suggested to tackle these problems, not the least of them being the proposal for an increase in interdisciplinary work with more financial limitations attached to the ethical nature of the work, and to make ethical approval of research projects obligatory before results can be published. Investigations into the operation of ethics committees by various professional groups is sorely needed, and investigations into the teaching of ethics in professionals schools is also required if change is to be promoted in a structured manner. Certainly an increase in ethical awareness among the new young research professionals holds a promise of hope for the future (Arnold and Sherwen, 1986).

David Fox, in his nursing research textbook, describes a survey he undertook of the amount of space researchers allow for a discussion of ethical issues in their research textbooks, and he was not overly impressed (Fox, 1982). Kileen, reviewing chapters on ethics in standard nursing textbooks, found interesting variations in the amount of space given over to ethics . . . in some instances none at all (Kileen, 1986). Fortunately the picture is improving and there is an absolute increase in ethical awareness among health professionals, even if this is still not adequate enough. Efforts are being made to actively promote an ethical work environment in the last few years, as demonstrated by all the professional activities already mentioned. Attempts are also being made to try and measure the extent to which the recent increase in ethical awareness is influencing practice (Felton and Parson, 1987).

In view of the current position of research codes and ethical concerns in research circles, and given the obvious necessity for research to be done with children (they too deserve the best treatments that advances in nursing practice, based on research, can offer) it became important to re-examine the position held by the British Paediatric Association and many other child-orientated professionals, that disallowed non-therapeutic research with children. Research was needed into the nature of research with children both well and hospitalized. A re-evaluation of the research process with children was obviously required, and in 1986 the results of a major survey into this area of concern was published under the chairmanship of Professor Dunstan. The work stands as a major landmark in the debate concerning experimentation with children and is already positively influencing the direction of paediatric research (Nicholson, 1986).

Meanwhile research nurses started to write their own research guidelines. The Royal College of Nursing published guidelines in 1984, the American Nurses Association rewrote theirs and published a new version of guidelines in 1983, and Canadian nurses published their guidelines in 1972. Additionally, the specific nature of paediatric research has prompted several national and professional bodies, including the British Paediatric Association in 1980, the US Government in 1985 and the ICN in 1983, to single out for special review the ethical problems of research with children. For nurses involved in research with children the usual risk/benefit ratio which must hold for all human research subjects becomes even more accentuated.

Research with children should be done for one reason only, to benefit the child or in the case of non-therapeutic research, to benefit other children, provided the investigator has obtained the assent of any child over seven years of age and the consent of adolescents, not only parental consent. Italy, for example, has no age in law when a child can begin to give valid consent for treatment and even English law emphasizes that children can, and should, always be asked for consent to treatment, but that from the age of 16 a parental veto is no longer binding. The British Paediatric Association explains this well, emphasizing the nature of the child–parent relationship by saying: 'that parents and guardians should be considered as trustees of a child's interests, rather than as having rights over the child' (Nicholson, 1986). This obvious ruling concerning paediatric research is not so obvious in the context of conducting research in a large teaching hospital, where sometimes it is difficult to distinguish between the many motives for a particular child being selected as a research subject (McClowry, 1987). The child with a rare metabolic disorder may become part of an investigative study that will never directly help the child or, if the condition is extremely rare, any other child in the foreseeable future either. The researchers investigating the nature of the disorder are not really interested in that particular child, or indeed any actual children; they are interested in extending knowledge concerning a rare disorder. This is what some researchers refer to as 'curiosity research', which is very important in helping to build up a body of knowedge but often hard to justify clinically.

A lot of thought would have to go into planning such a research study to ensure minimal disruption of the child's routine by the research protocol. Certainly no amount of pain inflicted while taking blood samples would be permissible. In such a case, the benefits to the child population at large are too small to justify inflicting (additional) pain on a hapless child 'volunteer'. Just how ethical it might be to take blood samples from healthy children was investigated by a team of psychologists, who concluded that blood-taking entails minimal harm to children, and is therefore ethically permissible (Smith, 1985). This conclusion is somewhat surprising since a number of studies show that children are terrified of injections and needles. The London study conducted by Smith included careful preparation of the children and this may account for the perception that minimal harm was done to them. Some moral philosophers argue that non-therapeutic research with children is possible regardless of the minimal risks involved, on the basis that participation in research can be seen as a growing and learning experience for the children (Redmon, 1986). It is as well to remember, as already mentioned in connection with non-invasive developmental research, that what constitutes the disruption of a child's routine can vary enormously from child to child and researchers should not be surprised if even apparently non-invasive research, such as collection of urine samples, is seen as too much of an invasion of a child's (and sometimes parents') privacy.

Sick children do not have to acquiesce to become research subjects, and the degree of disruption or discomfort is determined by the child not the researcher or accompanying adult. If a child assents to take part in research and the parent consents, then it is imperative that they both understand that they can withdraw from the study at any time. But a child cannot understand that it can withdraw from a study unless it understands about the nature of volunteering, the nature of research (from a participatory point of view), and the nature of withdrawal from participation in a study. The basic principle of ethical research, that it be conducted with volunteers who give free consent and with understanding of what is asked of them, still needs examination in the light of the knowledge we have about child development.

If informed consent is to be valid certain criteria need to be met and, bearing in mind our most vulnerable patients, these criteria deserve careful analysis. Much work has been done on determining levels of competency in order to be able to give valid consent for treatment and participation in research studies (Culver *et al*, 1980; Erickson, 1987; Roth *et al*, 1977). In order for the consent to be valid it is suggested that the following criteria to determine competency be present:

1. Evidence of a choice being made by the patient;
2. A reasonable outcome for that choice;
3. Evidence of 'rational' thought in making the choice;
4. Comprehension of the risks, benefits and alternatives.

(after Nicholson, 1986, p. 146).

Children when giving their consent to treatment or research are bound by these criteria just as adults are. The work of Weithorn and Campbell demonstrates that children can give valid consent. Their work with children tends to support the proposition that given the right help children can make reasonable choices concerning treatment and participation in research. (Weithorn, 1982; 1983). The single most talked about ethical issue in the research relationships with children concerns the extent to which children can give consent to treatment and assent to being used as research subjects (Leiken and Cound, 1983; Nitschke, 1982; Schowalter *et al*, 1973).

The debate, not surprisingly, centres around new levels of understanding concerning theories of child development, starting with the works of Piaget on moral development through to the works of Kohlberg (Piaget, 1969; Kohlberg, 1976; Puska, 1975). What is emerging is a systematic picture of children consistently applying cognitive and social skills to moral situations in a predictive fashion. In otherwords, moral development follows predictable milestones, similarly to social, physical and cognitive development. Thus, in Kohlberg's pre-conventional stage (where conventional refers to conventional conformity to rules) seven- to eight-year-olds can start to reason and comprehend moral issues, albeit haphazardly. By the time a child reaches 10–11 years this is fairly well established and all 14 year-olds (coinciding with puberty) can form conventional ethical reasoning. Here an appreciation of the welfare of others is beginning to be firmly established and altruism can start to be identified as a moral behaviour. At around 14 through to 18 years of age, a post-conventional moral stage may occur. This stage, however, may not occur in every individual. In fact some moral developmentalists would say not all adults achieve the highest stages of moral development, just as not all adults can be said to be content and self-actualizing in a Maslowian image of the life cycle.

Two identifiable stages at which children can be consulted have been selected based on these stages of moral development. Children can be approached for assent from the age of seven, that is the start of pre-conventional thinking, and at age 14 a youngster can give as reasoned a consent to treatment and/or research status as an adult (Nicholson, 1986). Nicholson found that the legal issues raised by the need for demonstration of competency to give consent, are not dissimilar to those found in studies concerning vulnerable adults. In Weithorn's study, a group of 14-year-old children demonstrated the competencies necessary to make rational decisions. In the study children from the age of 14 could make intelligent choices and decisions that compared favourably with adult decisions, and on parameters of 'reasonable outcome' nine-year-olds were as competent as adults. Similar findings of the rationality of young children and teenagers have been made by Leiken, Cound and Nitscke.

In order to demonstrate the competencies enlisted in Piaget's terms, formal operational thought processes are required, and since these skills can be carried out by a child of 11 years and over, and certainly by the time the child has reached the age of 14, perhaps health-care workers need to re-examine some of their ideas concerning 'age of reason'. Social scientists and health researchers are increasingly coming to the conclusion that it is lack of experience and information alone that is handicapping children in making rational choices and, as many a nurse can testify, the child that is unfortunate enough to have the requisite experience and knowledge of hospitalization is often more informed concerning his or her treatment choices than the average adult. Whatever legitimate criticisms may be levelled at the concept of 'informed consent', and many criticisms have been made, as far as children are concerned these same criticisms will hold. The meaningfulness of the exercise is as equally valid when it is conducted with children as with adults. Finally, the legality of research with children is still very hazy and nursing research would do well to heed the quote attributed to Edmund Burke:

It is not what a lawyer tells me I may do, but what humanity, reason and justice tell me I ought to do.

Although in the early part of this century children were cared for with their mother present and with a lot of stimulation (and fresh air), the low status of the paediatric nurse meant that the field of paediatrics became medically dominated with a paternalistic approach to health-care. This paternalistic approach precluded the idea of asking parents (or nurses) for permission to conduct research, obtain consent, disclose findings on participants, etc. No-one talked about informed consent or confidentiality, or the possibility of withdrawing from treatment or involvement in a research study. The morality of any single piece of investigative work rested on the individual integrity of the physician, social scientist and occasionally nurse, with predictably varying results.

In view of all these arguments we can now see how complex the issue of informed consent in children can be and how tortuous the long social and medical history behind the recent recommendations concerning research with children had become. It is now recommended that children too young to give a rational assent to involvement in a study, i.e. those under the age of six or seven, should also have their parents consent to participate in research. Since one person can only take moral responsibility for another in a very limited sense, in situations where a child cannot even assent to participate in research, only therapeutic or non-invasive research of minimal risk should be conducted. The parent giving full consent would, of course, be subject to the same competency criteria as would the child if it could consent. Should the child not wish to participate in the study, or to continue, e.g. to be so upset having to micturate on request for a urine specimen that he or she is having repeated bouts of anger verging on temper tantrums, then the child's wishes (however transient and infantile to the understanding of an adult) should be respected. Not to respect the wishes of a child would violate the second principle of ethical research. As Paul Ramsey explains – voluntariness and consent typify the rule of fidelity which demonstrates a level of minimum loyalty to children, since to experiment on children in ways that are not related to them as patients is already a sanitized form of barbarism (Ramsey, 1970). A child must be allowed to withdraw from a study by those who gave consent for the child to participate in the first instance, should the child be showing signs of stress or anxiety. A child's word is as valid as that of an adult; anything short of this touches upon that bugbear of modern health-care ethics – paternalism. If a child gave its assent or an adolescent its consent to be part of a research study, they too should be reminded that they can always withdraw from participating in a study.

I will not elaborate here on the need to eliminate all identifiable risks from a research study, although I appreciate that it is not always an easy concept to come to terms with in clinical practice (Richards, 1987; Bracken, 1987). By way of tribute to all nurse researchers who undertake participant observation studies, especially those studies that are also opportunistic in nature I wish to recall the case of the Jewish paediatric nurses in the Warsaw Ghetto of 1942. In 1942, Jewish nurses working in the paediatric hospital of the Ghetto found themselves involved in one of the most unusual research projects ever to be conducted (Winick, 1979). Out of the misery of the calculated hunger-disease inflicted on the children of the Ghetto, an idea arose by the Jewish doctors working in the children's hospital to do some observational, descriptive, non-therapeutic research with children. In a situation where nothing could be done to stop the advance of the disease the hospital staff who themselves were suffering from hunger and deprivation were consulted and they agreed to undertake to study the children in order to determine and describe the effects of end-stage hunger-disease on the health of these malnourished children. The nurses carried out their own psycho-social studies in addition to the studies for the physicians. Ultimately the study was smuggled out of the Ghetto, and the findings were subsequently published in Paris, later in post-war Poland and most recently translated and re-edited by Myron Winick for the Concepts in Nutrition Series of Wiley and Sons.

The obvious lack of informed consent in this unique instance is excused only by the fact that these children became unwittingly the sole possible subjects for the documentation of a disease process that in no other situation could ever have been clinically brought about or tolerated without intervention. The dying children of the Ghetto contributed to the understanding of the effects of hunger in children in a memorable way for which present day children suffering from hunger can only but benefit. This type of research brings out very clearly the moral duty to conduct opportunistic research when it is possible, for much that is of research interest could never be staged ethically. Researchers conducting such a study have an even greater obligation than usual to publish the results of the study (Reed-Ash, 1985; Warwick and Pettigrew, 1983; Bergman, 1984). The fourth principle for ethical research is that the benefits of the study should outweigh the risk to the subject. In cases of opportunistic research looking at effects of catastrophic events in the life of children, terminal disease processes, etc., the only ethical way around such an ethical recommendation is to make sure that the results of the study are widely publicized – that is, that the unorthodoxy of the research data or even research methods, is salvaged by the beneficial effects that the results of the study may have for subsequent children in similar circumstances. Naturally, where possible, even opportunistic research must follow known ethical guidelines. A nurse investigating the emotional benefits to parents of consenting to donate organs for transplantation from their child who has died from a road traffic accident, although conducting a form of opportunistic research, must ensure that his or her research methods and general approach to the subject are entirely ethical.

The question of who is qualified to do research is not easy to answer, since one could legitimately argue that only research carried out by full-time doctorally prepared researchers has any professional merit. In the UK, that would leave a very small number of research nurses interested in conducting paediatric research and capable of carrying out a research project. Most nurse researchers are educationalists, teachers or practice-based professionals. They combine practice, teaching or administrative work with research. The spirit of the last principle means that all research should pass through a peer review process and/or an ethics committee – it should be conducted by university trained nurses (who may also be staff nurses or nurse teachers but who have access to, or are working with, a qualified research mentor – and that the level of their work is of professional quality. The work should be open to professional scrutiny and criticism, which is usually a good control mechanism to protect the profession from inadequate research. Work that is unprofessional is a waste of time – and the ethical considerations of time wastage in the health-care field are worthy of some serious thought. Not only is wasting time and energy a travesty of the principle of justice – it can also violate the patient's basic right to be part of a worthwhile research study. Unprofessional research is demeaning of the integrity of the research subjects.

One way that patients can be actively protected from physical injury and/or emotional harm due to taking part in a research study is to help in the elimination of all possible extraneous risks involved with the study: all the nurses on a ward or in the community where the research is being conducted should acquaint themselves with the research protocol to the extent that the staff nurses understand the nature of the study and what may be the negative effects, if any, to that extent they will be in a better position to clarify matters with the patients who might have questions, and reduce their anxiety if need be. This approach is more likely to result in better data collection and therefore more meaningful results for the researcher. The response to the call for more interdisciplinary work will not only bring nurse researchers in closer contact with other researchers, which will broaden their outlook on different research methods, but hopefully the nurse's presence on the multi-disciplinary research team will contribute to a greater awareness of the ethical obligations that researchers have towards their patients (Nicholson, 1986). The interdependence of health-care professionals has wide implications for nurse researchers and nursing staff, as it is clear that no-one can stand on the moral sidelines while a patient is a research subject, even if that research is conducted by a professional from another discipline.

Nurses studying the efficacy of different types of mouth care for neutropenic oncology patients can be extremely intrusive into the child's private space. For most children, cleaning teeth twice a day is an inexplicable burden rarely understood by adults. For a child to be asked to clean his or her teeth and rinse his or her mouth several times a day using a special technique and then to record this, may be asking an awful lot of a sick child who even when feeling well would not enjoy the task of cleaning its teeth. The research, however, will probably help the children taking part in the research, and should certainly tell parents and paediatric nurses something about oral hygiene needs of neutropenic children. If the research design is scientifically sound, the research proposal should get a favourable hearing by the ethics committee.

It might be that one of the group of children in the study rinses their mouths with pure water after every meal, while another group of children rinses their mouths with an antifungal agent and medicated mouthwastes. Certainly if it were known what type of mouth care results in the least growth of pathogenic organisms, this would be of immense importance to nursing staff. For one group no attempt is made to actually prevent the growth of oral pathogens, except for the rinsing of the mouth with coloured water. What are the ethical issues involved in trials like this and can they always be justified? Does it make a substantial difference whether or not the patient is aware what mouth care treatment they are using? If the patient does not know whether or not he or she is actually rinsing his mouth with some special anti-fungal agent, because of deliberate research deception – what are the ethical issues now? Does consent to partake in research, even beneficial therapeutic research include consent to be deceived? We can argue that even children using placebo mouthwashes are better off than those not in the study, that is those in the control group, because this group actually rinse their mouth several times a day, albeit with water, compared to the control group of children who only clean their teeth twice a day. Apart from the questions concerned with the ethics of the study due to the research methods used, there still remain two areas of ethical concern. First, the justice involved in selection criteria to be used in the study for the randomization of patients, and secondly the problem of deception, addressed by many a social scientist over the past few decades. Anthropologists have had to grapple with the problem of deception for a long time. Margaret Mead expressed the

social scientist's viewpoint when she said: 'Beside the ethical consequences that flow from the contempt for other human beings, there
are other consequences – such as increased selective insensitivity or
delusions of grandeur and omnipotence – that may in time seriously
interfere with the very thing which he has been attempting to
protect: the integrity of his scientific work (Mead, 1970).

The problem, however, is not always due to the nature of the
researcher, as when a research nurse assumes the characteristics of
a difficult mother to study student nurses' reactions to such parents.
The deception can be in the form of built-in dishonesty in the very
research design of the form of concealment of the true nature of the
study, or some form of deception concerning the known variables
that the participants are working with. Mead again states that
secrecy in research violates the conventions of privacy and human
dignity and casts scientists in the role of spies, intelligence agents,
Peeping Toms and versions of Big Brother (Mead, 1970). Some
researchers would say that this is inevitable in some forms of
research, others that if research consent was validly given all would
subsequently be forgiven, while others at the end of the day, if the
true nature of the study is revealed, say that there will be no real
(or do they mean permanent?) deception. Sissela Bok, in her
excellent exposé of the nature of lying – looking at the ethical issues
involved in veracity and fidelity and the moral consequences of
breaking these principles – has much to say about lying in a medical
context and the use of placebos. Sissela Bok is not the only moral
philosopher to pick issues with researchers over deception, but her
clarity of scholarship make her writings almost compulsive reading
for the researcher interested in the problem of deception.

The ethics involved in using placebos in medical and research
studies centre on the violation of a person's integrity, since their use
can be devastating to the research subject. Ironically, almost all
information that a researcher could want can be obtained in an
honest, open way, and the only place left for a placebo might be in
the investigation of a drug where the trial calls for a double-blind
test of a pharmaceutical product where one of the medications
offered is in fact an inert sugar pill. The patients taking part in such
a study understand that they may in fact not be receiving a drug that
has known pharmacological effects, but then the researcher is no
wiser about the true nature of the drug either: all are equally
deceived. Such studies are rarely initiated by nurses, but certainly

nurses often have to administer the drugs. Understanding the nature of these trials is an aid to giving consent to be part of the research team, and no nurse should be part of a study unless he or she fully understands the principles involved. It is to dispel this research myth of secrecy that Mead said: 'wanting to know, when what one wants to know is valued by those from whom one must learn it, is an appeal that few human beings can resist – whether it is a desire to know how they trap game, how they pray to their ancestors or how many of their children have got second teeth' (Mead, 1970).

In conclusion, the paediatric research nurse working with children is under the same ethical constraints as his or her non-paediatric research colleagues. There are some research concerns unique to paediatrics, or of an increased significance in paediatrics, that researchers should be aware of, e.g. the significance of over-utilization of particular populations of children, the long-term effects that participation in research studies, especially longitudinal studies, can have on the research population. The effect of research participation on non-participant siblings is also a concern and the effect on parents of participating in research is not clearly understood (Jacobson and Straker, 1982; Zinzin and Goldstein, 1975; Simeonsson and McHale, 1981 and Showers and McCleary, 1984). The paediatric research nurse must abide by the ethical codes set down by her profession and even more than her non-paediatric colleagues allow herself to be humbled and awed in the presence of her patient-research subjects. Children embody the living natural example of how knowledge is gained, used and disseminated. Learning from children should take on a special significance for the paediatric nurse researcher, as the study takes on the characteristics of a shared adventure together with the children, mindful of the message that Pope John Paul II gave to the International Congress of Physicians and Surgeons in 1980

You must commit yourselves to a re-personalization of medicine. This means adopting a more unitary view of the patient and then establishing a more fully human relationship with him . . .. The relationship must become again an authentic encounter of two free human beings or as it has been put, between 'trust' and 'conscience'.

(Pope John Paul II, 1980).

REFERENCES

Arnold, J.M. and Sherwen, L.N. (1986) Belief Systems which influence research in nursing: Implications for Preparing future investigators. *J. Nurs. Educ.*, **25** (8), 325–7.

Bergman, R. (1984) Omissions in Nursing Research. *Int. Nurs. Rev.*, 1984, **31** (2) 55–6.

Bracken, M.B. (1987) Clinical trials and acceptance of uncertainty. *Br. Med. J.*, **294** (6580) 1111–2.

Carney, B. (1987) Bone marrow transplantation: nurses and physicians' perceptions of informed consent. *Cancer Nursing*, **10** (5) 252–9.

Clendening, L. (ed.) (1942) *Source Book of Medical History*. Dover Publications Inc., New York.

Culver, C.M. *et al* (1980) ECT and Special Problems of Informed Consent. *Am. J. Psychiatry*, **137** (5), 586–91.

Douglas, S. *et al* (1986) There's more to informed consent than information. *Focus on Critical Care*, **3** (2) 43–7.

Eisere, C. *et al* (1983) Children's knowledge of health and illness: implications for health education. *Child: Care, health and development*, **9**, 285–92.

Erickson, S. (1987) Gray areas: informed consent in paediatric and comatose adult patients. *Heart and Lung*, **16** (3) 323–5.

Feeny, P. (1964) *The Fight Against Leprosy*. American Leprosy Missions, New York, p 53.

Felton, G.M. and Parson, M.A. (1987) The impact of nursing education on ethical/moral decision making. *J. Nurs. Educ.*, **26** (1), 7–10.

Fowler, M.D. (1987) Voluntariness. *Heart and Lung*, **16** (1) 102–5.

Fox, D.J. (1982) Developing an ethical framework and protecting human rights. In *Fundamentals of Research in Nursing*, Appleton-Century-Crofts, Norwalk, Conn, pp 53–74.

Hodges, R.E. and Bean, W.B. (1972) The Use of Prisoners for Medical Research. In *Experimentation with Human Beings* (ed. J. Katz), Russel Sage Foundation, New York.

Jacobsen, R.S. and Straker, G. (1982) Selected methodological problems in research in child abuse: a developmental perspective. *Child: care, health and development*, **8**, 219–25.

Karani, D. and Wiltshaw, E. (1986) How well informed? *Cancer Nursing*, **99** (5) 239–42.

Killeen, M.L. (1986) Nursing fundamentals texts: Where's the ethics? *J. Nurs. Educ.*, **125** (8) 224–40.

Kohlberg, L. (1986) Moral stages and moralization, the cognitive-developmental approach. In Lickona, T. (ed.) *Moral Development and Behaviour Theory: Research and Social Issues*. Holt Reinhart and Winston, New York. pp. 31–53.

Leiken, S.L. and Cound, K. (1983) Therapeutic choices by children with cancer (letter). *J. Pediatri.*, **103** (1) 167.

McClowry, S.G. (1987) Research and treatment: ethical distinctions related to the care of the child. *J. Pediatr. Nurs.*, **2** (1) 23–9.

Melia, K. (1986) Informed consent – dangerous . . . *Nursing Times*, **82** (21), 27.

Mead, M. (1970) Research with Human Beings: A model derived from anthropological field practice. In Freund, P. *Experimentation with Human Subjects*, Braziller, New York, pp 152–77.

Nicholson, R. (ed.) (1986) *Medical Research with Children: Ethics, Law and Practice*. Oxford University Press, Oxford.

Nitschke, R. *et al* (1982) Therapeutic choices made by patients with endstage cancer. *J. Pediatr.*, **101** (3) 471–6.

Noble, M.A. (1985) Written informed consent: closing the door to clinical research. *Nursing Outlook*, **33** (6), 292–3.

Piaget, J. (1932) *Moral Judgement of the Child*. Routledge and Kegan Paul, London.

Piaget, J. and Inhelder, B. (1958) *The Growth of Logical Thinking from Childhood to Adolescence*. Routledge and Kegan Paul, London.

Pollock, L. and Tilley, S. (1987) *Why do nurses go to ethics of medical research committees? Decisions, experiences and reflections of novice researchers*. Paper presented at the International Nursing Research Congress, Edinburgh, Scotland.

Pope John Paul II (1980, Oct 27) Address to Congress of Physicians and Surgeons. *The Church Documents Quarterly*, **26**, (1).

Ramsey, P. (1970) *The Patient as Person*, Consent as a Canon of Loyalty, Children in Medical Investigations. Yale University Press, New Haven, pp 1–40.

Redmon, R.B. (1986) How children can be respected as 'ends' yet still be used as subjects in non-therapeutic research. *J. Med. Ethics*, **12**, 77–82.

Reed-Ash, C. (1985) Why nursing research? *Cancer Nursing*, Editorial, **8** (4) 1–17.

Richards, T. (1987) Exploring therapeutic risks (Conference report). *Br. Med. J.*, **294** (6588) 1678–9.

Robb, S.S. (1983) Beware the 'informed consent'. *Nursing Research*, **32**, 132.

Robinson, R.J. (1987) Ethics committees and research in children. *Br. Med. J.*, **294** (6582) 1243–4.

Roth, L.H. *et al* (1977) Tests of competency to consent to treatment. *Amer. J. Psychiatry*, **134** (3) 279–84.

Rothrock, J.C. (1985) Ethics committees, *J. Amer. Operating Room Nurses*, **41** (3) 527–8.

Shaw, A. (1973) Dilemmas of informed consent in children. *Eng. J. Med.*, **289** (17) 885–90.

Shelp, E.E. and Frost, N. (1980) Practising procedures on dying children. *Hastings Center Report*, **10** (4) 11–2.

Schowalter, J.E. *et al* (1973) The adolescent patient's decision to die. *Pediatrics*, **51** (1), 97–103.

Showers, J. and McCleary, J. (1984) Research on twins: implications for parenting. *Child: care, health and development*, **10**, 391–404.

Simeonsson, R.J. and McHale, S.M. (1981) Review: Research on handicapped children: sibling relationships. *Child: care, health and development*, **7**, 153–71.

Silva, M.C. and Sorrell, J.M. (1984) Factors influencing comprehension of information for informed consent: ethical implications for nursing research. *Int. J. Nurs. Studies*, **21** (4), 233–40.

Smith, M. (1985) Taking blood from children causes no more than minimal harm. *J. Med. Ethics*, **11** (3) 127–32.

Tornbjerg, and Jacobsen, L. (1986) Violation of human rights and the nursing profession. *Int. Nurs. Rev.*, **33** (1) 6–9.

Warwick, D.P. and Pettigrew, F. (1983) Toward ethical guidelines for policy research *The Hastings Center Report*, (Special supplement: *Ethics and Social Inquiry*) pp 9–16.

Weithorn, L.A. and Campbell, S.B. (1982) The competency of children and adolescents to make informed treatment decisions. *Child Development*, **53**, 1589–98.

Winick, M. (ed.) (1979) *Hunger Disease* (Studies by the Jewish physicians in the Warsaw Ghetto) translated from Polish by Osmos, M., *Current Concepts in Nutrition*, **17**, Wiley and Sons, New York.

Zinkin, P. and Goldstein, H. (1975) Ethical aspects of epidemiological studies. *Child: care, health and development*, **1**, 107–12.

FURTHER READING

ANA American Nurses Association (1985), *Human Rights Guidelines for Nurses in Clinical and Other Research*. ANA Publications D-46, Kansas City, MO. pp 1–16.

Australian College of Paediatrics Council (1981), ACPC Report on the ethics of research in children. *Australian Paediatr. J.*, **17**, 162.

Bartholome, W.G. (1977) Ordinary risks of childhood (letter). *Hastings Center Report*, **7** (2) 4.

Bok, S. (1974) The ethics of giving placebos. *Sci. Am.*, **231**, 17–23.

Bok, S. (1978) *Lying, Moral Choice in Public and Private Life*. Vintage Books, New York.

BPA (1980) British Paediatic Association, Guidelines to aid ethical committees considering research involving children. *Arch. Dis. Childh.*, 55 (1) 75-7.

BPA (1980) British Paediatric Association (Editorial), Risks and Benefits in Research on Children. *Arch. Dis. Childh.*, 55 (1) 2.

Broome, M.E. and Hellier, A.P. School Age children's fears of medical experiences. *Iss. Comp. Pediatr. Nurs.*, 10987, 10, 77-86.

CNA (1972) Canadian Nurses Association: Code of Ethics in Nursing Research. *The Canadian Nurse*, 68 (9) 23-5.

Davies, A.J. (1979) Ethical issues in nursing research: The National Commission for the Protection of Human Subjects. *Western J. Nurs. Res.*, 1, 324-6.

Davies, A.J. (1984) Ethical issues in nursing research. *Western J. Nurs. Res.*, 6 (2), 251-2.

DHHS (1979) *National Commission for the Protection of Human Subjects of Biomedical and Behavioural Research*, The Belmont Report: ethical principles and guidelines for the Protection of Subjects of Research, DHSS Publications, US Government Printing Office, Washington, DC.

DHHS (1983) Additional protections for children involved as subjects in research (45CFR46). *Federal Register*, 48, 9814-20.

Downs, S.F. and Fleming, J.W. (1979) Issues related to Human Subjects. In *Issues in Nursing Research*, Appleton-Century-Croft, New York, pp 107-49.

Duska, R. and Whelan, M. (1975) *Moral Development: A guide to Piaget and Kohlberg*. Paulist Press, New York.

Foucault, M. (1973) *The Birth of the Clinic: An archeology of medical perception*. Translation by Sheridan, A.M. Tavistock, London.

Goodwin, J.S. (1979) Knowledge and use of placebos by head officers and nurses. *Ann. Intern. Med.*, 91 (1) 106-10.

Holm, K. and Llewellyn, J.G. (1986) *Nursing Research for Nursing Practice, Practical considerations in the ethics of Human Investigation*. W.B. Saunders, Philadelphia, pp 229-44.

Katz, J. (1972) *Experimentation with Human Subjects*. Russell Sage Foundation, New York, chapters 8, 11 and 12.

Lynn, M.R. (1986) Children have rights too. *J. Pediatr. Nurs.*, 1 (5) 345-8.

Mahon, K.A. and Fowler, M.D. (1979) Moral development and clinical decision-making. *Nursing Clinics of North America*, 14 (1) 3-12.

Mitchell, K. (1984) Protecting children's rights during research. *Pediatr. Nurs.*, 9-10.

Moore, I.M. (1982) Nontherapeutic Research Using Children as Subjects. *MCN*, 7 (5) 285-94.

Pearn, J. (1987) A classification of clinical paediatric research with analysis of related ethical themes. *J. Med. Ethics*, 3, 26-30.

RCN (1977) *Royal College of Nursing: Ethics related to Research in*

Nursing. RCN, London.

RCP (Royal College of Physicians) (1986) Research on healthy volunteers. *J. of the RCP of London*, **20** (4), Special groups: children.

Rodin, J. (1983) *Will this Hurt?* Research monograph, Royal College of Nursing, London.

Shrock, R. (1984) Moral Issues in Nursing Research. In Cormack, D.F.S. (ed.) (1984) *The Research Process in Nursing*, Blackwell Scientific Publications, Oxford, pp 193–207.

US Government (1947) *Nuremberg Military Tribunals, Trials of War Criminals.* US Government Printing Office, Washington, DC.

Warnock, M. (1985) *A Question of Life – The Warnock Report on Human Fertilization and Embryology.* Blackwell, Oxford.

Watson, A. (1982) Informed consent of special subjects. *Nursing Research*, **31** (1) 43–7.

Weinreich, H. (1975) Kohlberg and Piaget: Aspects of their relationship in the field of moral development. *J. Moral Educ.*, **74** (3) 201–13.

WMA (World Medical Association) (1964) *Declaration of Helsinki Recommendations Guiding Doctors in Clinical Research.* WMA, New York.

Appendix A
International Council of Nurses, Code for Nurses: ethical concepts applied to nursing, 1973

The fundamental responsibility of the nurse is fourfold: to promote health, to prevent illness, to restore health and to alleviate suffering.

The need for nursing is universal. Inherent in nursing is respect for life, dignity and rights of man. It is unrestricted by considerations of nationality, race, creed, colour, age, sex, politics or social status.

Nurses render health services to the individual, the family and the community and coordinate their services with those of related groups.

NURSES AND PEOPLE

The nurse's primary responsibility is to those people who require nursing care.

The nurse, in providing care, promotes an environment in which the values, customs and spiritual beliefs of the individual are respected.

The nurse holds in confidence personal information and uses judgement in sharing this information.

NURSES AND PRACTICE

The nurse carries personal responsibility for nursing practice and for maintaining competence by continual learning.

The nurse maintains the highest standards of nursing care possible within the reality of a specific situation.

The nurse uses judgement in relation to individual competence when accepting and delegating responsibilities.

The nurse when acting in a professional capacity should at all times maintain standards of personal conduct which reflect credit upon the profession.

NURSES AND SOCIETY

The nurse shares with other citizens the responsibility for initiating and supporting action to meet the health and social needs of the public.

NURSES AND CO-WORKERS

The nurse sustains a cooperative relationship with co-workers in nursing and other fields.

The nurse takes appropriate action to safeguard the individual when his care is endangered by a co-worker or any other person.

NURSES AND THE PROFESSION

The nurse plays the major role in determining and implementing desirable standards of nursing practice and nursing education.

The nurse is active in developing a core of professional knowledge.

The nurse, acting through the professional organization, participates in establishing and maintaining equitable social and economic working conditions in nursing.

Reproduced with permission of the International Council of Nurses.

Appendix B
UKCC Code of Professional Conduct for the Nurse, Midwife and Health Visitor, 2nd edn, 1984

Each registered nurse, midwife and health visitor shall act, at all times, in such a manner as to justify public trust and confidence, to uphold and enhance the good standing and reputation of the profession, to serve the interests of society, and above all to safeguard the interests of individual patients and clients.

Each registered nurse, midwife and health visitor is accountable for his or her practice, and in the exercise of professional accountability shall:

1. Act always in such a way as to promote and safeguard the well being and interests of patients/clients.
2. Ensure that no action or omission on his/her part or within his/her sphere of influence is detrimental to the condition or safety of patients/clients.
3. Take every reasonable opportunity to maintain and improve professional knowledge and competence.
4. Acknowledge any limitations of competence and refuse in such cases to accept delegated functions without first having received instruction in regard to those functions and having been assessed as competent.
5. Work in a collaborative and co-opertive manner with other health care professionals and recognise and respect their particular contributions within the health care team.
6. Take account of the customs, values and spiritual beliefs of patients/clients.
7. Make known to an appropriate person or authority any conscientious objection which may be relevant to professional practice.
8. Avoid any abuse of the privileged relationship which exists with patients/clinets and of the privileged access allowed to their property, residence or workplace.
9. Respect confidential information obtained in the course of professional practice and refrain from disclosing such information without the consent of the patient/client, or a person entitled to act on his/her behalf, except where disclosure is required by law or by the order of

a court or is necessary in the public interest.

10. Have regard to the environment of care and its physical, psychological and social effects on patients/clients, and also to the adequacy of resources, and make known to appropriate persons or authorities any circumstances which could place patients/clients in jeopardy or which militate against safe standards of practice.

11. Have regard to the workload of and the pressures on professional colleagues and subordinates and take appropriate action if these are seen to be such as to constitute abuse of the individual practitioner and/or to jeopardise safe standards of practice.

12. In the context of the individual's own knowledge, experience, and sphere of authority, assist peers and subordinates to develop professional competence in accordance with their needs.

13. Refuse to accept any gift, favour or hospitality which might be interpreted as seeking to exert undue influence to obtain preferential consideration.

14. Avoid the use of professional qualifications in the promotion of commercial products in order not to compromise the independence of professional judgement on which patients/clients rely.

Reproduced with permission of the United Kingdom Central Council for Nursing, Midwifery and Health Visiting.

Appendix C
United Nations Declaration of the Rights of the Child

PREAMBLE

Whereas the peoples of the United Nations have, in the Charter, reaffirmed their faith in fundamental human rights, and in the dignity and worth of the human person, and have determined to promote social progress and better standards of life in larger freedom.

Whereas the United Nations has, in the Universal Declaration of Human Rights, proclaimed that everyone is entitled to all the rights and freedoms set forth therein, without distinction of any kind, such as race, color, sex, language, religion, political or other opinion, national or social origin, property, birth or other status.

Whereas the child, by reason of his physical and mental immaturity, needs special safeguards and care, including appropriate legal protection, before as well as after birth.

Whereas the need for such special safeguards has been stated in the Geneva Declaration of the Rights of the Child in 1924, and recognized in the Universal Declaration of Human Rights and in the statutes of specialized agencies and international organizations concerned with the welfare of children.

Whereas mankind owes to the child the best it has to give.

NOW THEREFORE THE GENERAL ASSEMBLY PROCLAIMS

This Declaration of the Rights of the Child to the end that he may have a happy childhood and enjoy for his own good and for the good of society the rights and freedoms herein set forth, and calls upon parents, upon men and women as individuals and upon voluntary organizations, local authorities and national governments to recognize these rights and strive for their observance by legislative and other measures progressively taken in accordance with the following principles:

Principle 1

The child shall enjoy all the rights set forth in this Declaration. All children, without any exception whatsoever, shall be entitled to these rights, without distinction or discrimination on account of race, color, sex, language, religion, political or other opinion, national or social origin, property, birth or other status, whether of himself or of his family.

Principle 2

The child shall enjoy special protection, and shall be given opportunites and facilities, by law and by other means, to enable him to develop physically, mentally, morally, spiritually and socially in a healthy and normal manner and in conditions of freedom and dignity. In the enactment of laws for this purpose the best interests of the child shall be the paramount consideration.

Principle 3

The child shall be entitled from his birth to a name and a nationality.

Principle 4

The child shall enjoy the benefits of social security. He shall be entitled to grow and develop in health, to this end special care and protection shall be provided both to him and to his mother, including adequate pre-natal and post-natal care. The child shall have the right to adequate nutrition, housing, recreation and medical services.

Principle 5

The child who is physically, mentally or socially handicapped shall be given the special treatment, education and care required by his particular condition.

Principle 6

The child, for the full and harmonious development of his personality, needs love and understanding. He shall, wherever possible, grow in the care and under the responsibility of his parents, and in any case in an atmosphere of affection and of moral and maternal security; a child of tender years shall not, save in exceptional circumstances, be separated from his mother. Society and the public authorities shall have the duty to extend particular care to children without a family and to those without adequate means of support. Payment of state and other assistance towards the maintenance of children of large families is desirable.

Principle 7

The child is entitled to receive education, which shall be free and compulsory, at least in the elementary stages. He shall be given an education which will promote his general culture, and enable him on a basis of equal opportunity to develop his abilities, his individual judgment, and his sense of moral and social responsibility, and to become a useful member of society.

The best interests of the child shall be the guiding principle of those responsible for his education and guidance; that responsibility lies in the first place with his parents.

The child shall have full opportunity for play and recreation, which shall be directed to the same purpose as education, society and the public authorities shall endeavour to promote the enjoyment of this right.

Principle 8

The child shall in all circumstances be among the first to receive protection and relief.

Principle 9

The child shall be protected against all forms of neglect, cruelty and exploitation. He shall not be the subject of traffic, in any form.

The child shall not be admitted to employment before an appropriate minimum age, he shall in no case be caused or permitted to engage in any occupation or employment which would prejudice his health or education, or interfere with his physical, mental or moral development.

Principle 10

The child shall be protected from practices which may foster racial, religious and any other form of discrimination. He shall be brought up in a spirit of understanding, tolerance, friendship among peoples, peace and universal brotherhood and in full consciousness that his energy and talents should be devoted to the service of his fellow man.

Reproduced with permission of UNICEF.

Appendix D
NAWCH Charter for Children in Hospital

1. Children shall be admitted to hospital only if the care they require cannot be equally well provided at home or on a day basis.
2. Children in hospital shall have the right to have their parents with them at all times provided this is in the best interest of the child. Accommodation should therefore be offered to all parents, and they should be helped and encouraged to stay. In order to share in the care of their child, parents should be fully informed about ward routine and their active participation encouraged.
3. Children and/or their parents shall have the right to information appropriate to age and understanding.
4. Children and/or their parents shall have the right to informed participation in all decisions involving their health care. Every child shall be protected from unnecessary medical treatment and steps taken to mitigate physical or emotional distress.
5. Children shall be treated with tact and understanding and at all times their privacy shall be respected.
6. Children shall enjoy the care of appropriately trained staff, fully aware of the physical and emotional needs of each age group.
7. Children shall be able to wear their own clothes and have their own personal possessions.
8. Children shall be cared for with other children to the same age group.
9. Children shall be in an environment furnished and equipped to meet their requirements, and which conforms to recognised standards of safety and supervision.
10. Children shall have full opportunity for play, recreation and education suited to their age and condition.

Reproduced with permission from NAWCH, National Association for the Welfare of Children in Hospital, Argyle House, 29–31 Euston Road, London, NW1 2SD. Telephone 01-833 2041.

THE ICN DECLARATION ON NURSING RESEARCH

Nursing research

The International Council of Nurses is convinced of the importance of nursing research as a major contribution to meeting the health and welfare needs of people. The continuous and rapid scientific developments in a changing world highlight the need for research as a means of identifying new knowledge, improving professional education and practice and effectively utilizing resources.

ICN believes that nursing research should be socially relevant. It should look to the future while drawing on the past and being concerned with the present.

Nursing research should include both that which relates to a total research plan and that which may be undertaken independently. In nursing research available resources of different levels of sophistication should be utilized and research should comply with accepted ethical standards. Research findings should be widely disseminated and their utilization and implementation encouraged when appropriate.

ICN believes that nurses should initiate and carry out research in areas specific to nursing and collaborate with related professions in research on other aspects of health. Nursing research should involve nurses practising in the area under study.

National nurses associations are urged to promote the development and utilization of nursing research in cooperation with other interested groups.

Guidelines on nursing research for national nurses associations

Nurses associations can contribute to the development and the quality of nursing education and nursing service by promoting nursing research in their countries. The human and material resources as well as the scope of involvement in this effort vary from country to country. Therefore the following guidelines are presented as possible avenues for action which need to be adapted to the local scene by the nurses association.

Organizational framework

The establishment of a nursing research group within the association can provide a basis for determining association policy and action on nursing research. Such a group may take various forms such as a research committee, a section of nurse researchers, a research foundation.

This group may include nurse researchers, nurses in the various fields of nursing service and nursing education, and other qualified persons who can enrich the group.

Functions

Education. The association should promote an appreciation and understanding of research and the preparation of nurse researchers. Inclusion of a research component in basic and post-basic nursing education programmes, workshops, study days and other media may contribute to the achievement of this aim.

Coordination. The association should explore and develop channels for coordination and cooperation with other groups concerned with nursing and health related research such as government agencies, professional organizations, educational institutions, research institutes, foundations and other non-governmental agencies.

Survey. In cooperation with other groups, the association should survey the scope and direction of completed and on-going research. This overview could be used to identify gaps and overlaps in order to set priorities for future projects.

Master plan. The association may participate in the development of a long-term master plan which could serve as a guide to researchers in the selection of projects and for the allocation of resources. However, such a master plan should not inhibit creative interests and efforts that fall outside the plan.

Facilitation. The association may facilitate research among its members by identifying and/or providing, where possible, guidance, consultation, funds and other resources. A forum for discussion of on-going research may offer guidances and encouragement to researchers. The association may encourage the creation or development of a system of information concerning completed nursing research in that country.

Dissemination. The association should encourage the distribution of research findings and implementation of the recommendations when appropriate.

Adopted by the Council of National Representatives of the International Council of Nurses, Tokyo, Japan, May 1977.
Reproduced with permission of the International Council of Nurses.

Appendix F

RCN Society of Paediatric Nursing. Statement of values in paediatric nursing

---

The child is a unique developing individual.

The family is the significant group of people who are the child's primary support group in his life, i.e. parent(s), foster parent(s), guardian, siblings or others.

The paediatric nurse has a responsibility for children in relation to the promotion of health, the prevention of illness, the restoration of health and the alleviation of suffering. S/he is accountable to the child, the parents, him/herself and the statutory body.

The environment should protect and facilitate the child's growth and development.

The child refers to any individual from birth through to adolescence.

The paediatric nurse refers to an individual with the appropriate qualification for nursing children.

We subscribe to the United National Declaration of the Rights of the Child 1959 and to the National Association for the Welfare of Children Charter for Children in Hospital 1984.

The child has a right to give and receive information about himself appropriate to his stage of development.

The health care of children should be planned in such a way that the integrity of the family unit is maintained.

The perceptions and expectations of the family in terms of the need for health care should be carefully ascertained and incorporated into the nursing care plan.

The physical, mental, emotional, spiritual and social needs of parents should also be considered, particularly in relation to the well-being of the child.

If a conflict of interests arises between parents and child, the vulnerability of the child requires that the nurse gives priority to his/her need for natural development, health and well-being.

As paediatric nurses we have a particular concern for the protection of children who are not yet autonomous individuals in law. We are governed furthermore by the UKCC Code of Professional Conduct which requires each registered nurse to safeguard the interests of individual patients and clients.

With sensitivity and imagination the nurse should attempt to view the world through the child's eyes. S/he should encourage the child to express his opinions and concerns.

The nurse should fulfil an advocacy role in interpreting the needs of the child where necessary to other members of the health care team.

The paediatric nurse should be aware of trends in society which may threaten the health and well-being of children, and should fulfil an advocacy role where necessary to the wider public.

Where nursing care is provided by the nurse in the child's home, s/he should promote an awareness of health hazards.

Where hospital care is necessary, the nurse should ensure an environment which is safe and which will minimise the potentially damaging effects of stress and separation.

August 1987.

RCN, 20 Cavendish Square, London, W1M 0AB.

Index

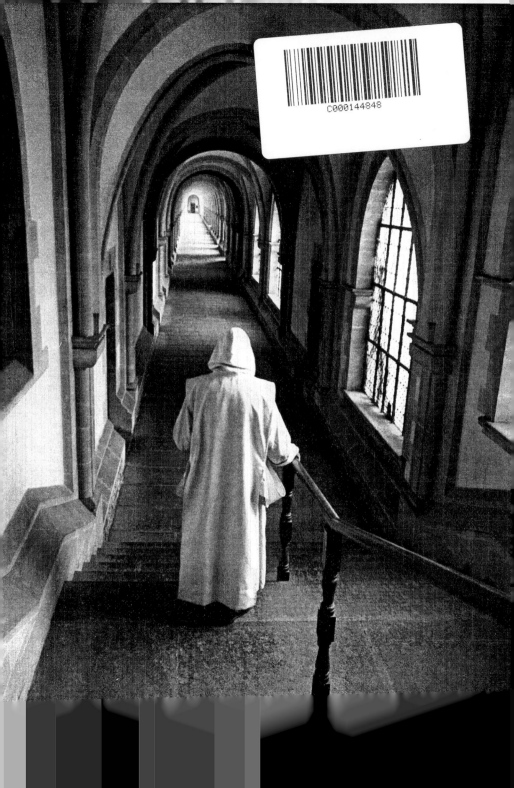

"O Bonitas!"

A Glance from the Heart

Speaking's deadweight in the silent world of God.
A Word suffices for the architect of thought,
A glance of love for Uncreated Love.
God's a new world, a world of shorthand: Love
Is he and Love his language. No laboured style,
No ocean of ink, no volumes of endless type.
Not even a whisper is heard in the heart of God
Where all his children sing an ecstatic song
In silence
Of timeless adoration. Love the fount
Of Being floods in everlasting speech
A Word beyond articulation, the Act
Of Being, Jesus forever clothed in Flames.
The Pillar of Fire, God's inward joy and bond,
Creates our hearts receptive, a single lyre,
For God's eternal Voice: the Breath of Life.
Loving says all in the silent world of God ...

For Robin N. Bruce Lockhart, Apostle of Silence

"O Bonitas!"

Hushed to Silence

A Selection of Poems
by a
Carthusian Monk

chosen by

Robin Bruce Lockhart
(author of *Halfway to Heaven* and *Listening to Silence)*

GRACEWING

First Published 2001

Gracewing
2 Southern Avenue
Leominster
Herefordshire HR6 0QF

Front Cover St Hugh's Charterhouse, Parkminster
(photo: Johnathan Winstanley 1960)

Reverse part title page The Little Cloister, St Hugh's Charterhouse, Parkminster (photo: Bob Collins)

Back cover Communion at the Chartreuse
Monks chanting the Office at the Grande Chartreuse
(photos: Robin Bruce Lockhart)

ISBN 0-85244-550-4

Printed & bound by Antony Rowe Ltd, Eastbourne

CONTENTS

vi

INTRODUCTION

Life has its ups and downs but the one big "up" in my life has been the ability I have had to visit nearly every Charterhouse in the world and to meet Carthusians of many nationalities and backgrounds. That this came about was due to a few days retreat I made many years ago to the English Charterhouse at Parkminster in Sussex, where I truly met God face to face. Coming to terms with this took a good many years but the ultimate result was my book *HALFWAY TO HEAVEN* – an expression St. Thomas More once used to express his feelings when he attended night office at the London Charterhouse.

The Carthusian Order was founded by St. Bruno in 1084 and of all the Saints he is certainly the one who deserves the epithet 'Great'. Bruno thirsted for God alone and to return to that life of prayer and devotion in silence and solitude which Our Lord had inspired in the early Christians and, in particular, the Desert Fathers. Bruno's ideal of renouncing the world for prayer and penance in silent solitude so that there was no room for anything else in the soul but God has been faithfully followed by the Carthusians down the centuries. In the words of Pope Pius XI: "The Carthusians have so well preserved the spirit of their Founder, Father and Lawgiver that, unlike other religious bodies, their Order has never in so long a space of time needed any amendment or, as they say, reform".

For about 40 years now, I have had a remarkably close and privileged relationship with the Carthusians. Because – rather than despite – of their contemplative life of silence and solitude, I have never met such happy men and women (there are Charterhouses for women). One of the Carthusian mottos is: To make saints not to publicize them" and when I am within the walls of a Carthusian enclosure the breath of God seems to emanate not only from the monks and nuns but from every cell, every flagstone and every blade of grass. In the words of St. Bruno: "Only experience reveals what benefits the solitude and silence of the desert bring to those who have it." And, to quote from Pope John Paul II's message to the Carthusians on the 900th anniversary of their foundation: "It is not so important what you do, but what you are. This seems to apply in a special way to you who are withdrawn from what is called the active life."

The Carthusian day begins when much of the world is carousing or just starting to sleep off the excesses of a materialistic day. At 11.45 pm, the monk rises from his bed to say the Little Office of Our Lady. Leaving his cell, he winds his way through the cloisters to the monastery church. The choir stalls fill up, the professed monks in their white habits, the novices in their black cloaks. The church is in almost total darkness. The only light comes from the sanctuary lamp and the shaded low lamps in the choir. After deep silence, the chanting of the long night vigil of Matins and Lauds begins. The chanting carries in its cadences soaring praises of God, then sinks to low supplication. It seems to break into sobbing repentance, a holiness all its own. And as the sung Office proceeds, it is impossible not to sense how the fervour of the Psalms takes over.

The purity of the Carthusian chant has been zealousy maintained for centuries; it is slower, lower-pitched and less melismatic than the Benedictine chant. The 17th century Cardinal Bona, who undertook vast research into liturgy, records that it was the Carthusian chant which Christ recommended in revelations to St. Bridget, the patron saint of Sweden. No instrument accompanies the chant.

The Carthusian Mass, devoid of pomp and ceremony, closely resembles the old rite which Charlemagne obtained from Rome in the 8th century. It has been little changed in a thousand years. A Carthusian will spend time prostrate during Mass, as a meaningful act of adoration at the consecration of the body and blood of our Lord.

A DAY IN THE LIFE OF A CARTHUSIAN FATHER IS AS FOLLOWS:

11.45	Rise
Midnight	Little Office of Our Lady
12.15 am	Matins/Lauds (in church)
2.45 am	Little Office of Our Lady (in cell). Sleep
6.45 am	Rise
7.00 am	Little Office of Our Lady. Prime (in cell)
7.30 am	Spiritual Exercises in cell
8.00 am	Little Office of Our Lady. Terce (in cell)
8.15 am	Conventual Mass (in church)

10.00 am	Spiritual Exercises (in cell)
11.15 am	Little Office of Our Lady. Sext (in cell)
11.30 am	Dinner (in cell)
12.30 pm	Relaxation. Cleaning of Cell, mending etc
1.15 pm	Little Office of Our Lady. Nones (in cell)
1.30 pm	Spiritual Exercises (in cell); also, perhaps, some gardening
3.30 pm	Little Office of Our Lady (in cell)
3.45 pm	Vespers (in church)
6.45 pm	Angelus (in cell)
7.15 pm	Compline (in cell)
8.00 pm	Sleep

On Sundays and solemn feast days, the timetable is somewhat different and on Mondays, the Fathers leave their enclosure and go for a three hour walk in the countryside and break silence to converse with each other.

The Brothers, who opt not to be ordained, care for the material needs of their Charterhouses, spending some seven hours a day out of their cells, which until relatively recently consisted of just one room, but now tend to be similar to the cells of the Fathers. They see to the preparation and cooking of food, look after the vegetable gardens, deal with general maintenance and the cutting up of firewood. A Brother prays silently while at work, which is almost always carried out in solitude and for the most part in silence. Every year, each Brother makes a 'retreat' and remains in the peace and solitude of his cell for eight days. On Sundays and solemn feast days a Brother will remain in his cell for most of the day in contemplation. Today, the lives of Fathers and Brothers are more integrated than at any time in the Order's history.

Thinking about the numerous Fathers and Brothers I have met in the Order, I found the variety of their backgrounds not only fascinating but illuminating: soldier, artist, hunter, farmer, singer, cinema owner, heir to an Empire, a jockey. Once integrated in the Order they were all as one, so to speak. Many may have brought crafts with them into their Charterhouses but some had exceedingly great artistic talents of a nature which I would describe as gifts from God and reflecting what the French philosopher Jacques Maritain would – I paraphrase – describe as attributes of one of the unlimited sides to God – Beauty.

I have heard some outstanding singing from a Carthusian, wonderful paintings by another, very fine silverworkmanship and writing. I have, at Parkminster, also discovered a poet whose work I and others outside the Order consider to be some of the finest poetry in the English language written in the twentieth century. I found out, little by little that he has written nearly 1,000 poems – most of which he has never shown to anyone. I persuaded him to let me read them all and from these I have selected about 100 poems to give some idea both of the beauty of his inspired creativity but also its variety. Much that Carthusians write remains in their archives. I think it of great importance that at least these 80 poems should be printed and made permanently available in libraries everywhere.

Feast of the Exaltation of the Holy Cross, 2000

Robin Bruce Lockhart

Our Secret

Through silent cloisters I walk and sense You near.
The world grows paltry and dull, its anxious care.
This our honey dripping upon the hills
Our wine unstinting poured, our manna strong;
Your love, our secret; our wealth, this wilderness.
No purpose beyond these walls, my heart's for this:
To enter this love of God exceeding great,
To know it and thirst for more; to seek it and grow
In depths of longing. Through summer warmth I walk
And icy wintry days; through war and peace;
Through building and eviction; expanding swift,
And failure; through life's misfortunes, phases, laws
I walk as many have walked these very stones
So much they longed for God, his will, his peace.
Men stay convinced You spoke their name, are found
Within as Truth, experienced as strength of will
No name can indicate. Life's purpose unlocks
All force and virtue beyond poor earthly hopes;
Hopes of fathomless depth: O the Mystery of God!

Labour By Candlelight

Warm candlelight
Falling as faith gives fire to the Sacred Word;
While night with ineffectual force
Raids this hallowed sphere.
Here I sit and ponder
And feel at one with thousands
Of whom the world knew nought,
Who down the ages did as I do:

Lived by candlelight
Falling night by night;
By loving trust turned words to holy wonder;
Struck flames from the Sacred Rock,
Burned to be with God as I do ...

Untitled

Circling your holy altar with frankincense,
(Our urgent intercessions and ardent sighs)
Our Chalice speaks to me, significance
So rich in broad and welcome lip, in size:
Your image, silent central, adored in state.
The Song of Songs comes swirling uncontrolled,
Its gems of truth flash, intoxicate:
Its imagery is living here so bold
And mystic, elusive silver as festal sign;
Cup of wedded love in symbol discerned.
"Drink deep O Lovers! Drink my Blood as wine,
My life, atrocious death; my Heart has earned
    In violence to see your face in vision. Taste
    My hell, my heaven: my cup run not to waste!"

Saviour

Saviour sleeping in my bark,
Silently you guide me through the dark.
I must not look to the land I've left,
Nor to the sea, nor to the sky,
But look at you, Saviour, where-you—lie.

Saviour sleeping in my heart,
Secretly you pierce me with that dart
Of aching exile, of paining you.
And though to eye and ear concealed,
Deep calls to deep for the heart must be revealed.

Saviour sleeping in my soul,
Splendidly reveal that intimate role
Your holy wisdom has shaped me for,
Enlightening my eyes to see one spark
Of infinite Love sleeping in my bark.

Departure

I would depart and go to Paradise.
The Lord has called and what can keep me here?
The world no longer smiles nor can entice;
My work is done and death holds nought to fear
For One has borne my sins in sacrifice.

O come with me, my Friends, to Paradise!
I loath to leave you here in Shadowland,
Though you are good, it's true, and no device
Of Satan can allure you from his hand
Who planted you like fires on floating ice.

Still follow soon, my Friends, to Paradise!
O come grey earth and matchlight of the sky!
O come pale moon and myriad eyes of mice!
The childhood days are passed, the shadows fly,
The perfect comes, the Prince, our Paradise!

Transfiguration

What did you see, Peter, on the hilltop?
What man longs to see, feels it should be
Christ shot through with splendour,
In his true world wrapped in glory.

What did you hear, James, upon the hilltop?
Heard faith's pioneer, Lord and Master;
Prophets call him Saviour,
Majestic voice resound like thunder.

What did you plan, John, upon the hilltop?
Planned to live for mankind's vast salvation,
A world shot through with splendour,
Christ each soul's transfiguration.

What shall we see, Jesus, on the hilltop?
What God longs to see, Bride made holy,
Spouse shot through with splendour
In my Heart, wrapped in my glory!

Silence and the Psalms

A clap outside my window, or blackbird's wings
Flapping through the torpid afternoon?
Whichever it broke the silence and left me more
Of quiet to concentrate my heart, distil
More love on the psalms. Delight as masculine
As David's whose heart is psalmody, an isle
In a sea of wreckage. His heart of human things
Sounding across the years in a timeless tune
Invites my soul God's being to adore
Beyond the beyond or close in this daffodil,
All present within my grasp, present within
These psalms which God to sinners reconciles.
    O God, my soul's that clap in a magnitude
    Of silence, your loving mercy's infinitude!

The Snowdrop

In the ruins of a stone built shed
A snowdrop grew
And no one saw.
Each year it bloomed
Each year it died
And no one saw.

O tiny flower,
What power there is in beauty!
Fear not for being small.
I breathe in beauty's power
And I am more.
And no one saw.

No one?
O Snowdrop.
The silence cracks?
The stones that shelter you.
O snow-white petals
Plunged in awesome sight!
O tiny stamen,
O magic wand
That fills the galaxies
With eyes of light!

Isaac

Father Abraham,
Walk with me,
The two of us together.
Willingly I bear the faggots
And the fire;
Willingly be bound
And laid upon the stones.
Father, lift up the knife!
I would be sacrificed as he was,
Rise as he rose.
I would be prince where he is
King of Glory,
Holy as he is holy.
Father Abraham,
Walk with me in silence
The two of us together.
I would ascend the Mount of Providence
My hand in yours,
O Father of cast-iron faith!

Still Life

An open window:
Smoke hazy mountain
Deforested, aloof
Beyond the quilted plains;
Ink sketched poplars
Against a reddening sky;
A green flame of ivy
Clinging to the lichened stones;
A lone red rose;
A cowled figure diverts his eyes
Resumes the sacred text,
Sighs with lonely longing,
Flicks over the pages
In the twilight
Century after century ...

Red Tulips

When the fields are gay at morning
May I rejoice before you
Like red tulips.

When the fields with labour ring
Refresh my soul with silence
Like white snowdrops.

When the fields are cool at twilight
Imprint your wounds within me
Like blue violets.

When the fields are lost in night
Draw me where love's burning
Like dark roses.

Rosmini

Rosmini, master in thought and virtue, long
I've sought your guidance and saintly influence,
And now this touching act of friendship! A song
Of gratitude is due in recompense.
But more to please you: more zealous in each event;
A builder of Holy Church; discerning more
By prayerful waiting God's will as sacrament;
More hungry for your teaching than heretofore.

St Bruno, confirm my heart's determination:
To form one spirit with Jesus crucified;
To seek the Father's glory, the Spirit's unction;
And by your grace made humble and sanctified,
    To store up virtue by prayer more than before,
    And through Rosmini's wisdom to spill that store.

Six Rivers

Evil flows on the face of the earth
As blood flows from the heart of Christ;
    And who can staunch it?

Suffering flows on the face of the earth
As suffering tortured the heart of Christ;
    Who can endure it?

Death floods out on the face of the earth
As death did drown the heart of Christ,
    And who can end it?

Mercy flows from the heart of Christ
And inundates this world of ours;
    And who would staunch it?

Life springs forth from the heart of Christ
And sparkles over the face of the earth:
    Who can resist it?

Love bursts free from the heart of Christ
And turns all suffering to sacred bliss,
    And who would end it?

The Sonnet

Well pointed Sonnet in cadence, form and thought
Resolves a tangled twilight of rapier light
In tranquil, artistic peace; the vague is wrought.
This satisfaction, Beauty's Face, night
Enshrouds; moonstreaks in maddening gleams reveal.
So hacks the sonneteer through ancient boughs
And new shoots full of hope till he may kneel
In breathless expectancy (the Muse allows
Some respite): the fought for Face appears. He heaves
A sigh and counts his labours well repaid.
His eyelids weigh and sleep invades; he leaves
This world in peace for dreams where moonbeams raid.
    Truth and Beauty to wed: my grievous dream!
    My untamed shrew, Pure Holiness, redeem!

September Dawn

Copper glinting sun and darkened boughs,
And the leaves as bright as bottled wine. I fell
To praising overjoyed; to beauty bows
The peoples bewitched by this the morning spell.
The unvanquished pool of light with varied face
Shrugs off the night and claims earth's awed concern.
This ruthless god once cowed our ancient race
And though no more in dread yet still we turn:
Beauty was made for man and man for song.
Beauties of time may play us false, still
Who want may yet revere the Artist. Prolong
Your hymn, O Mary, of gratitude, the thrill
Of the heart's spontaneous joy in God's design:
The beauty of 'good' is Love's true fingersign.

The Cross
The form
Of Love
Is still
A King dead upon a hill.
Oh what is Love that yet does kill!
So fierce
In bloom:
That Love
Which
broke
The tomb!

Time and History

Time seems ruthless;
History aimless.
Time though plays a part,
History hides a heart.
A Heart of unrepented scars.

A Giant that links the earth and stars.
And he is marching in his might,
A flaming pillar wrapped in night.
He crushes prince and power disarms,
Yet lifts the lowly in his arms.
And he will take them swiftly where
The stars are gambolling in his hair:

Fear not the march of time
Nor history full of crime.
Faith reveals God's plan:
Love in the Son of Man.

A Paradise of Heart

Come, Seraphim with flaming swords, turn
All futile thoughts from out my mind, burn
All vain desires from out my heart! I call
On you, my God, to rectify my fall,
      To make my mind a Paradise all through
      Where you may walk and I may worship you!

What joy to know you, to know you created me;
What joy to own the Incarnation, to see
The Cross as truth, to revere the love that bore
This death for me. What joy when we adore.
      O make my mind a Paradise all through
      Where you may walk and I may worship you!

A silent temple, words all held in peace,
A breathless awe, a watchful love increase;
A tranquil confidence that I shall find
This temple secure within my grateful mind.
      O make my mind a Paradise all through
      Where you may walk and I may worship you!

And will you ever read these words again,
Or let them wash your heart like the pounding rain
Washes the shining sand of futile weeds?
For the pound of eternal waves how my shore bleeds!
      O make my mind a Paradise all through
      Where you may walk and I may worship you!

A Paradise of heart is where God dwells
And there his pleasure finds. When the curfew knells
May I not hide in shame. In confidence
May I approach newborn to innocence.
      O that my heart were a Paradise all through
      Where you may walk and I may worship you!

Dream River

Love is a movement, a glimpse of a star,
Love is a song shining with zeal,
Power in the heart and boldness of view.
Love is a thrush unstopped of its song,
A tumbling of notes irrepressibly borne
Through twilight of day and the loneliest hour
With night on the wing and her lover is dead.

Love is a river shot through with the sun
Flowing through jewelbeds of ruby and pearl,
Running unchecked on its silent advance
To the tumult of waters, adventurous sea.
O River of dreams, hypnotic and deep,
I sleep by your banks attentive in peace:
For I know that the River is Saviour and God.

The Height

We walked together across the ferny heath
Exchanging simple or holy thoughts. The trees
Of beech were parasols at times beneath
The noonday heat. The Height appeared. The breeze,
A mercy; the southern Downs so far away,
A vision worth the climb. So easily swayed
By nature's heroic scenes you gazed while gay
The clouds passed by their part in silence played.
The Height, its beauties are locked in memory. (O time
Chameleon concept; an ache, a jewel, a wall!)
These priceless moments when we our earthly climb
Is done may we, in mercy clothed, recall.
    O Mary, unite us now and in God's sight
    Who walk together in faith a mystic Height!

Standards of Sorrow

Orwell took a pessimistic stance.
Eliot too; but there's a difference.
Orwell's town was tiny.
Eliot's City was large as heaven.
A difference of dimension,
One insignificant, one absolute:
Standards of compassion.

Orwell saw his town walls crumbling,
Night encircling,
Tyrants triumph,
And he was sad.
Saw people dying wholesale,
Lose their tiny life,
And he sadly mused.
Saw an age die like pigs
And like them were no more.
And if some persons were great
And he admired them,
They too went their way
And Orwell shed one tear.

Eliot saw men not just dying
Saw them living dead.

Not lose their tiny life
But lose the incalculable life
Christ cast on the earth like fire.
Man's fall's no minor thing,
Mere fall of a Golden Age.
He saw a world abandon
Mystic peaks of hope;
Descending
To wastelands of atheistic savagery.
Nor did it make him sad:
Niagran tears flooded down his face,

He tore his hair
And screamed across the moon …

Christus

By night he leapt
Down from the sky
  To childhood.

On earth he grew
In grace and power
  To Manhood.

By sympathy
He learned of vic-
  timhood.

Then we through pride
Killed him misun-
  derstood.

Dying he grew
To love as no
  Man could.

Rising he raised
A priestly Brot-
  herhood.

Ode to a Snowflake

Snowflake settling upon my fingertip,
I'd raise a monument to your name before
My hot blood destroys your fragile beauty, the warmth
Of life prove deadly, completes your destiny.

Yet words, to what avail are they? This heap
Of unhewn stones thrown down like a rugged cairn
Will stand to mark your momentary dance
Of death, frail Snow Queen's debut and destiny.

Art, sublimer than fact, is fingersign,
Voice of the heart, prophet of Gospel peace;
Yearnings for beauty shaped in the searching mind:
Enduring snowflake, glimmerings of destiny.

The Silence of Eden

Adam! My son!
Can you not hear me call?
I heard your footstep fall.
Adam! Adam!
Can you not hear me calling?
Do crickets chirp so loud,
Or night owls screech so long;
Do lions growl so strong,
Does thunder fill the cloud?
Is their not silence falling?
Adam! Adam!
You cannot hear me call:
Nights thunders round your fall.
O Adam, my son!

Wisdom and the Way to Peace

Wisdom in sovereign adoration flows
Through silence her dark pavilion: this sacred world
Of truth where all is said by giving. The heart
Is untranslated, undiminished gift,
Is unrestrained and outright: Love only loves.
Our loving's shade of that great Rock; a tale
Not fact; a tantalizing vision. Our hearts
May brush yet pass on as stars in orbit. We love
But in desire: we may not knit as one.
Our hearts still gaze in silence and lover's hope.
    O Wisdom and the way to peace!

Wisdom appeared as hope grew pure of eye.
Hope outgazed all bitterness; beyond
All tragedies ignoring the brutal scene
She gazed; of war and deportation; of death
(So final so fearsome, so dense that prophets failed
To see beyond it and centuries passed in fear
Or fatalism or half-denial); beyond
This hideous giant she gazed and drank her power
On one profound conviction: God's granite love.
She gazed as children gaze in solemn peace.
    O Wisdom and the way to peace!

Waste and void where Wisdom broods. Waste
And Word creates. "That he would kiss me!" Bride
In vision cries, "Come, Lord Jesus! Come!"
Intensity and depth of Scripture! One faith,
One voice, from Waste to Song to Rushing wind,
Fusing Babel's long-abandoned Tower
In Symboled speech: hope's genesis in tongues
Of praise round Mary's pondering Heart. Here all
Her children fly, gazelles that leap for joy,
While Wisdom in sovereign adoration flows.
    O Wisdom and the way to peace!

In the Beginning

Reflecting its light amid the fluttering leaves,
The stained glass windows of the woods, the dark
Cathedrals of the world. Here loving hands
Reach up to the sun and touch its beams.
They feel the warm light streaming from above,
Are joyful to behold this world that teems:
The sand about the sea, the furry peach,
The velvet mole and all the sun makes bright
Reveal the Maker's tenderness and teach
His detailed foresight and inaccessible light.

Cascading cries the blackbird,
Joyful sings the lark;
And shy the nightingale
Goes piping through the dark;
I can hear the woodpie
Tapping on the bark,
And sparrows twittering gaily
Scrapping in the park.
The cuckoo in the distant
Woods has found his mark;
The bird of Paradise
Is singing, let us hark!

Pillars of Light

O Lord,
Among the stars,
Who-is-life,
Gave me Life,
Drenched
My eyelids with stars,
My locks
With the drops of the night,
Sent me down to give
Mortals
Life
Abundantly
Among the stars.
And the columns
Of dust
Shone
With terrifying
Light,
Shattered
In fear,
Dis
integrated,
New born
As living galaxies,
A symphony,
A Rose,
A song of joy
Sweet
Like honey
Dropping in the heart,
Loud like thunder,
Like the sound of many
Waters:
"Holy! Holy! Holy! ..."

Where do Sunsets Go?

Where do they go? I've watched them curtsy low
In tender gold and blushing pass from sight.
I've seen flamingo silence sinking slow
Beneath the sea and cried that lonesome night.
Oh where do heartbreak sunsets go? I stilled
My heart till understanding came. All die
Resisting death their latent treasurer spilled
With pure extravagance along the sky
To shimmer from their grave, the deep dread sea.
Oh evil waste! What anguish to watch my wraith
Expelled from its ruined home! Adam's decree!
How could we face all that except in faith?
    Your sunset, Saviour, spelt dawn for all that dies:
    Where weeping mortals go immortals rise!

Bluebells

O Bluebells, O whispering bluebells,
Spilled on the sheltering wooded pass,
Lowly angels who praise prolong
Hushed in adoration's love unseen.
O summer sky adrift at Eastlands,
Bluebells, shimmering bluebells!
    Cool, dim, twilight blue; chime-like
Your name is music, O bluebells!
Soft-blue, magic carpet of EastLands,
Poor-folk's beauty, their song to heaven's Queen.
My tears sparkle with your song!
O the pain of beauty: you sing and alas,
Then vanish ... O whispering bluebells!

Graves of God

O Graves of God,
Live stones of faith!
Spires of hope
That pierce the sullen skies,
Draw earthwards promised fire:
New life born of God!

Sin like a festering flower
Died in the death of God.
God/Man was raised by God:
All are raised in power!

I see the grave and Christ ascending,
The empty tomb and mercy pending;
And in the Blood of sacrifice
Resplendent the spires of Paradise!

The Clock

A clock once hung upon the wall,
Made little noise but told the time;
    It was esteemed by all.

But then one day it lost its face
And told the time no more. It lost
    Its meaning, lost its place.

It was well made all did agree
But what it was and why it was
    Was not so plain to see.

Aesthetes ungrudging their tribute paid,
"A thing of beauty's a joy for all,"
    But more was not betrayed.

It made utilitarians pall:
Devoid of use it stood condemned;
    It had no rights at all.

But scientists were really sold;
They filled vast libraries with its laws:
    Its purpose was manifold

Morning and Light

And in that Face futility will flee,
The weight of failure resolve in joy.
O Morning Star, cast out the cruel "night"!
Let "night" soon be done
And all its empty, fleeting deeds.
Fill me with immense salvation
To spend in deeds of immortal value.
The fish-eyed vacancy of time,
The pointless to-fro swim of fashion,
Power and wealth; O tedius "night"!
The great blind ocean ruled by the Prince
Of Darkness holds thrall
The silver shoals, the children of Light.
St Peter, bless my vado piscari,
Make fruitful my futile "night";
Guide me stripped in zeal casting
In blind faith to rescue souls.
Then in the "morning" Jesus
Will beckon from the shore. No longer
Vado piscari; the nets are full
And in the Light glittering the catch
Will break our hearts with gladness!

Volcano

Volcano
Seething continually
In wonder and expectation;
Hungering to my hidden roots,
Hungering for that moment:
Eruption of my total power,
Eruption of my total structure,
Eruption of violent lava
Burning so deep, so long,
So violently; dissatisfied in time;
Eternity alone my mark.
O blind, burning lava,
Burst from time!
Flame from the deep roots!
Explode, destructive Power,
Extinct stars still glimmering
In memory's Pectolian depths.
Cleanse their light, O Lava,
White hot Spirit-grace,
Violent within my heart!
O Power incredible
Within this shell!
Fire of Love, my new life,
Live in this crumbling, dead
Volcano!

Swinging Sunsets

Sunsets studding a golden sky
For "All Saints". It fits the bill!
Great Saints, I love you! I magnify
Your brightness beyond the blood lined hill.

O Sacrament in festive mood,
Enkindle my slumbering spark,
My poor spent moonlight faith! O food
And symbol, strength while the roads are dark.

Swinging sunsets, Greek and Jew,
Dazzle the golden sky:
The Bridge if plain is golden through
Where Saints like sunsets multiply.

They cast an undiminished spell
Rejoicing the faithful throng.
Fair piece of cherry cake, farewell!
Symbol of saints and Bridal song,

Down to my hidden depths be wed
Hidden in a world apart,
Hidden as holy hunger, O Red
And golden Bride, humble my heart!

Penny Bright

The day's light stepping rays will not appear,
Nor lazy noonday shadows sleep. The hewn
Face of the sundial no shade shall trace, a clear
Reminder of things no longer opportune
When time has fled. No trumpet shall sound the fall
Of night; no lonely watchman turn his mind
(Distressed in starlight solitude) to all
His own, his sleeping children, wife and kind,
Nor linger on day's reconquest, silent, bright,
Unknown. No sleeper shall turn from dreams with sighs;
No soldier anticipate the brutal fight
Resumed: the war with evil's done. The eyes
    Of Christ have conquered. Joyful in God's flame
    His children, penny bright, sing to his Name!

Beneath Your Altar

Envious of the pure who wait beneath
Your altar of sacrifice (slain like you
But here till wrath so total rests in its sheath
And mercy triumphs they wait while all made new).
I weep with downcast eyes. Unworthy wretch
Am I to gaze on these so lovely, to hear
Their sweet complaint of eager longing. O stretch
Your hearts, grant me purer love! Fear
Is rightly mine till virtues bloom. What grace
I squander, largesse to the foulest. I ache to lie
Beneath this altar concealed in martyr's case
Impatient with the pure who call me on high.
      God's flesh drunk with vengeance flows with peace.
      God Triune visioned my anxious ravings cease!

Sun of Justice

A new Sun broke
Red on the hill and the light
Spilled over and down;
And the darkness scattered the rooks in fear
And the valley rose up gay.
And the dewdrops glistened on the Pilgrim's eyelids
As he stirred on the banks of the stream.
And his eyes glanced up to the hilltop far
And the Red Sun kindled his heart.
He reached for his staff
And his song was glad
As the pathway slipped behind.
And the Red Sun beckoned
And held his view. And he cast his burden
On the mountainside and he rose
With a lighter step; for the steep path
Glittered that once was dark and it lead
Where his heart was lost.
For it ran to the hilltop wrapped in Light
Through a wound in the Scarlet Sun ...

Peter The Tramp

Peter comes into our life
Twice a year perhaps as he
Circulates the South stopping
Mainly at religious houses.
Some give him gardening jobs
And pay, meals and a few nights rest up.
He attends their religious services,
Even the long Orthodox Easter which
Ended as he told me in a barbecue
At 3 am. He slept a few hours
Then set off again on his bicycle.
He looks truculent but is in fact
Very gentle and trustworthy. A Baptist
Orphanage reared him and he's kept
Its religious dispositions. He loves God
And asks questions about religious
Matters while I tend to his feet.
He gets blisters and never cuts his toenails.
I feel honoured to perform this humble
Mandatum. He says he loves to stop
On a hill and watch the sunrise and
Think of God. I know I am
In the presence of someone God loves.
I often think of his 'purpose' or 'witness'
In life. God leads him all round
The gentle South where he leaves a perfume
In the air: the sweet odour of Christ.
I weep as I write. How loveable he is,
Peter the tramp.

The Shore

Why am I loitering still here upon the shore
Between the sea and the land of Evermore,
When one invasion of the land would make it mine,
When all the hills invite me in to dine?

O Hamlet-heart of mine, do you still hesitate
Upon the shore by the sea and the land of fate?
O come then, strong decision, turn and take the land;
The valleys smile and touch your trembling hand.

The sea laps the shore, curls round my naked feet
And gently calls me to where the waters meet.
O Jesus, how vast the sea, how vast the waves of sin!
But all the trees cry out, "Haste within!"

Race Colours

Rest at pale evening;
A young slim tree,
Girl flowering tenderly
    Yellow like me.

Peace at pale morning;
A song set free,
Christ coming joyfully,
    White like me.

Work at new morning,
The blind must see,
Christ teaching powerfully,
    Ruddy like me.

Agony at lone evening;
A tall grim tree,
Christ bleeding wantonly
    Red like me.

Silence at dread evening;
Corpse on a tree;
Christ tasted hell for me:
    Dead like me.

Clouds at dark evening,
Thunder on the tree;
Christ comes majestically:
    Black like me.

Rest at bright morning,
Peace running free:
Go loving endlessly
    God-like me!

St Hugh's

I've found my home, my heart it fills;
Here men indwell the Burning Dove;
Here beats a bell that tolls for love,
St Hugh's crowning the Sussex hills.

No doubts have I: God calls me here,
Where hidden within his loving care,
He teaches me that love to share
With all mankind purchased so dear.

So lifelong within this charterhouse
My selfish heart I will redress
And serve my brothers with eagerness;
And fill with prayer my Father's house.

The world may fear this tiny cell
But all the world is held within
The Heart of Christ who bore our sin:
That Heart's our home, our citadel.

I hunger for nought but holiness,
The power of loving, the power to save,
The power to live beyond the grave
With him and his in happiness.

O Mary our Mother, Fount of Grace,
O Burning Bush and Lily Flower,
So guide us beyond this giddy hour
That we may see God face to face!

Savage Sunset

O Father, if I love not life
In you, nor to share Christ's death in you,
My heart's a charnel-house: and more,
    Death gnaws the heart.

No Christ, no Cross. No Cross, no life.
No vehement heart, no hope, no locks
Wet with the drops of the night; yet more,
    Death gnaws the heart.

O Savage Sunset, my dawn, my life,
My Paradise unbound, my Stag
Leaping upon the mountains; no more
    Death gnaws the heart!

My Anxious Art

Our words are like the waves upon the sea,
Rippling far from the shore.
Our words are but a surface,
Sounds that quiver and are no more.
    Bright Reapers, show my anxious eye
    Where angels gaze and children do not cry!

"My Word is hammer to smash the doors of bronze;
My Word is fire, is rock,
A living sword, two-edged,
True, guiding my wayward flock."
    Bright Reapers, show my anxious eye
    Where angels gaze and children do not cry!

How long, O foolish heart, this worthless game
Of rhyming! The night is past,
No longer self your prison,
Smashed in pieces what held you fast.
    Bright Reapers, show my anxious eye
    Where angels gaze and children do not cry!

The Death of Dom Stephen

O Place remote, denied to mortal view
Where Stephen's soul aspired, where angels vie
In adoration, where all is always new;
O Place so awesome, so far beyond our sky!
Yet Stephen has no dread. His childlike eyes
Seem blind to doubt or hesitation. They gaze
Beyond too simply for deception or lies
To cloud his hope: his Saviour will crown his days
Of faith. No anxious doubts may intervene;
Where love is perfect all fear is cast from sight.
His eyelids close. No more this earthly scene
Pervades his playful eyes now turned to Light.
    O Angels, goad me on to Heaven's shore
    A place more fair now Stephen's gone before.

Sky Over the Hill

Through the silence of solitude
Some walk searching for life; they sigh,
"O Bonitas!" Not sad their eye
Through loss but waiting, a ceaseless cry
Of longing, an ache for God. Divine
Who lingers briefly as Bread and Wine;
Enduring his holy Face will shine ...
O heart, how deeply I feel your sigh
To find with them beyond this sky
That light-year lingering beatitude!

The Seventh Tale

"Stop and consider!" cried the mournful youth,
Who tells us many a tale but not the truth.
The Seventh Tale was lost; he knew but six,
And they reflect this lower world that fix
The senses firm. But of the Heart that moves
The stars, informs the mind, the Heart that proves
The truth of all men do, he's nought to say.
Stop and consider! Life is but a day
Spent upon the summer Rose; the world
A dewdrop held in petals homewards hurled.
O Flaming Petals, of mortals spes unica;
O Rose of Sharon! O Rose of Golgotha!
    Poor Adonais, great melancholy Keats!
    Had he but known, what then his lyric feats!

Envied Termination

The brunt of centuries of persecution fell
On this man in whom no trace of worldly power
To brace our confidence resided; fell
And broke in cruelty unbridled. This hour
Was his, the hour of meekness and gentleness,
The hour of Prior Houghton maturing deep
In Christ and now revealing that blessedness.
His meed: a Christ-like death. The hangmen sweep
All dignity aside and disembowel
The priest holding his wrenched-out heart on high.
The alabaster jar, smashed with a scowl,
Still perfumes Tyburn still lingers in England's sky.
    "Verse, Fame and Beauty are intense indeed,
    But Death intenser: Death is Life's high meed."

The Empty Tomb

Have I come to this, an empty tomb,
With ointments to anoint Messiah, to pass
From hope to fear, to gaze into this gloom
And find no corpse to touch, no Lord alas,
For one to balm? And some did say a King
Was he; and Peter said he'd conquer all
The world as Alexander did. A King,
Like that! He trampled men like mud in all
His glory, streams of human blood but spittle
In his path: like that, a King! Oh Peter,
Did you draw so close and learn so little!
Jesus spoke our names, came from the Father;
    He loved all people, the sinful, poor and lowly,
    But they have murdered him who loved me! "Mary!"

The Pain of Nothingness

Plunging into pointlessness day
After day, diminishing to insignificance
In anguish (a straw swept on by the desert wind;
A cork on the frightning sea; a child lost
In a crowd startled by sudden glimpse of self,
His pain of panic and isolation, bewildered
Stares at the passers-by, seeks one form
Familiar, the hand he held, one face, one voice),
I walk in a world not mine, too big to possess,
    Too fleeting to understand.

Called into solitude, called by a voice
Familiar, held by a hand well known, led
To solitude's reverse, to fellowship,
To oneness with He-who-is, I walk in a world
Made mine. Inserted where heartbeats rise, where eyes
Startled behold the Face so longed-for, bewildered
Man finds himself. The world's too small for man:
O freedom from the small! The human heart's
A mystery too terrifying to plumb, a point
    Too God-close to understand.

Prodigal on Fire

Father, I cleave to you intensely, cling
In reverence, hope so passionately for peace
In spite of unvanquished self-indulgence! Wing
Me over sin's infested road! Increase
My cleaving to eagle's intensity! It sinks
Sharp talons of confidence like anchors. I crave
Your Face (my stymind sneers and lewdly winks)
O Father awaiting on the road so grave
In expectation this worthless son's return!
Begrimed so deep in selflove stypen stench
Envelops me; the more I seek you, yearn
For you, the more it suffocates. Drench
With waters clean my soul, deep its dye
Of bestial disregard for God. The pure
Who love unwounded soar like falcons. I sigh
Remembering them; their perfumes still mature.
Oh to devour this road! Irrepressible haste
Plucks my sinews, Father, to reach you; adore
My Saviour and his Gift of Splendour! On fire to taste
High torrents of peace and angels joy restore!

Rose Intangible

Sad is every poet.
Born to dream he knows
His dreams are stillborn. Rose
Intangible his dream; plucks it
By night rejoicing; rejects it
When dawn's clear light expose
The poet and his rose.
    Sad is every poet.

Grave is every poet.
Nightly there his keep
Where rosebuds awaking peep.
Kneeling he seeks to steal it,
Fresh in his heart to seal it.
Cruel day chucks it down,
Butt-end into the town:
    Grave is every poet.

Torn is every poet.
Joyful the muse of art;
No thought in music's dart;
My muse: to bridge all being,
A bird on chaos brooding.
Poetic forms ensue,
Enthrall: yet Love withdrew.
    Torn is every poet.

Lone is every poet
Resolving his inward storm
To fairest fragile form,
So rich, so clear, so living,
Grand Pyramid outliving.
O salvage and render just,
Jesus, my forms of dust!
    Lone is every poet.

God most strong

Fairy lights they seem to me the apples
Hanging on the trees; along by the wall
Strawberries are ripening while red tomatoes
Hymn the sun. Scarlet blossoms dot
The runners curtain of green and silken tassels
Grace the sharp blade maize. And can I smell
Potato fields in blossom? Lo! The dwindling
Sun has turned the corn to floods of gold!
How summer paints with fire and fruit and song!
Good earth lifts up its face to God Most Strong!

Son

Man, who from the first failed to reach
His goal, in time threw up one perfect Man
Who realized that goal and thus could teach
In life, in death, the quality of man.
God's Son by nature; ours by need: did we
Not cry for him, "Drop down dew, sweet sky!"
At last epitomized in him we see
Ourselves: our birth, our pain, our death; and high
Above the gibbet, behold, transfigured through,
Man enters God's domain. Our future lies
In him, in him salvation. So with our true
Self born anew we walk through parted skies.
     Lead on, Great Son of Man, our human goal;
     In life, in death, our resurrected soul!

Portrait of John

Meditation has made John deep and silent,
More prone to pondering the Word of God
Than preaching; yet preach he must. His conversation
Weaves a spell-like incantation. His thought
Flows diamond-clear and how his treasured memories
Quicken my heart! They vivify my hopes.
Each detail he recalls with awe as loving
Faith pursues Messiah's course and death,
Impressions which shaped his youthful understanding
Arresting his growth in worldliness; a child
Remaining simple in speech and deed; an eagle
In Christ-like penetration, divine in depth
Of vision, mature in love's demanding virtues.
Ecstatic his countenence when day by day
He breaks the Eucharistic Bread in mystery:
Silent together we live on the Flesh I bore ...

Epitaph To A Friend

One more candle quenched that played its part
And made the room congenial; one more bird
Is silent; one more vacancy in my heart:
My friend is dead. Our friendship is deferred.
You died but the work was done. Another came
With far more claim to friendship whose love you knew
Of old and longed for, who spoke your deepest name.
We root too deep features of mortal hue.
My friend is dead. I fear to touch the chair
He used; the ache returns. I glance away
Swift to deceive my heart. Moscini, I wear
Your memory like a millstone. All flowers decay
    Before me and visions of the summer pass:
    My friend is dead; he sleeps beneath the grass.

Colour Blind

By strange enabling we believe.
We see much more than sight reveals.
We see in colour, so to speak,
While others see but tints and shades.
This 'more' we must convey to them
Or live a lie to the truth. We must
Complete their lives, enrich their hearts.
Yet to express this 'colour' proves
Too much; people could never guess
Till shown: the rainbow still is grey
For them, its beauty has not flamed;
The sunset like a thunder storm
Sucked down the whirlpool of the West.
We speak that light splayed is hued
And men but smile. We self-exclude
Our lives from the stark grey world.
Our world's a blaze of spectral light.
Yet friends refuse to venture far
From homely things of grey. O cold,
Grey City, graveyard neat and clean!
May Turner's sun yet shine on you,
Spill its blood across your tombs,
Though men loved darkness more than light.

Hushed To Silence

A new kind of spring grows in my heart.
I feel hushed to silence
While the stage is being reset. Where
Are the stark trees gone and the cold, white sky?
Where's the monotony of a too long winter?
There is movement, colour and sound.
And there are new birds. Did they not migrate
Seven years ago? I told myself
They would not return, they had died
Over the ocean, they did not care. And there
Is warmth too forcing the bulbs
Into new life. Fresh green is hope.
Hope springs anew where there is love.
I must be in love always, hold hope
By the hand as dew sparkles in the sun.
I feel hushed to silence
As a new kind of spring grows in my heart ...

My Angel goes before me

Woe to those who scandalize me,
Behold no depths within me,
 My point,
 My ground of being.
O millstone of monstrous woe!

 My angel goes before me,
Beholds God's face continually;
He prays within me,
Adores with jubilant wing,
(O vast and awesome thing)
 My ground of being:
One mass of burning Divinity!

Love me seeing my dread totality,
 My point,
 My ground of being:
This fierce, consuming splendour!
 My angel goes before me ...

The Beautiful To Ponder

The Beautiful to ponder
As Mary ponders, merges eye
And mind to live in wonder.
In wonder's gaze we linger
And prize that more in vision; we sigh
Till loving blooms in hunger.

She ponders a new creation
Spring from deadwood, rise in power
From the spilled Blood. (O Wisdom,
Beauty's a priestly kingdom!)
In pangs her new child stirred: this Flower
Of the Spirit and compassion.

To ponder as Mary ponders
Renders eye and mind and heart
One soul where nothing sunders
This flower of Life. Wonders
Awake great depths of being, impart
Beauty for the love that ponders.

Prospero's Farewell

Our little life is rounded by a dream,
A dream which rose (before the tempest, before
The wreck) sublime in concept in Paradise;
A vision that maid's will see and old men dream,
A scheme of things repulsed but not destroyed,
A broken plan whose wintry face no more
Will appear when Spring investing Paradise
With innocence will reign in glory. O dream
Enshrined in a fallen race that blindly aimed
To build it on some hill, to place before
Its eyes, to touch the pain for Paradise
In the human heart. O heart, this mundane scheme
Has failed you along the aching years and mocked
To scorn your paltry monuments! Then soar,
Poor heart, so devious, unto Paradise
Now lit by immaculate day unending. That dream
Is worth the dreaming. Ten fathoms deep are drowned
My sins: my heart in sorrow hungers the more
To gaze with rapt attention on Paradise.
My little life, be rounded by this dream!

Mount Anathemata: The Savage Trophy

Hung on the battlements of heaven,
Hideous to exterior darkness,
These ultimate things devoted,
Objects of dread, deep wonder and exultation;
All citizens who sign their lips with freedom,
Dazed, eternally burn with veneration;
Corpse and Cross, plunged in desolation,
Love cut and murdered plumed humiliation,
Sin's cruel triumph, power and violation.
Ceaseless upon the battlements creation
Awed breaks out in myriad voices,
    Fired by jubilation:

"Power to Love all conquering! Heaven
Bow in joy exceeding! Darkness,
Cower! O Christ exalted,
Behold our gratitude, our exultation!
Stunned by Love's extent of pain (in freedom
Died for freedom, forgave sin's foul corruption),
We wake from death in tears of warm compunction.
O Savage Trophy, Rood of desecration,
Streaming suffering your phial of consecration!
O King and Prophet, Priest of all creation!
O Corpse and Cross, intense our voices
    Sing of our salvation!"

Wisdom and the way to peace

O dull sun, rise no more! This night is sun
And song for me, is rose and city pure!
O dead sun, gouge out my sordid eyes to star
Your Ghost Town's dome of fear! They gazed all day
In tears but did not see! It's night (this night)
They have in anguish unknowing sought! O strong
Immortal One, O Flames of Fire, my Blaze
Of heart, my understanding, my fortitude,
My vision vast and inexhaustible, my life,
My holiness (as yet not mine) my fear!
    O Wisdom and the way to peace!

Wisdom makes children speak and stones to sing:
"Hosanna! Son of David!" Our God who dwells
In silence has dawned in holy Flesh on hearts
That mourn in darkness where lethal shades encroach.
Silk eyelids, close! Seal out this two-faced Town
Sold to lies outright! Seal me within
This visioned world of symbols, this language I feel
At one with; it speaks so vividly, the heart
Of truth perceived (its flesh will decompose).
O Night exultant when sealed-up thunders speak!
    O Wisdom and the way to peace!

The Centurion

Surely this Man was innocent.
His dying was beautiful
Like slow, unfolding sunsets
Upon the sea. Teardrops they distil
But touch me not with envy.
I envy who die in God:
Sunsets as fair as innocent.

Godsong

That more be given (outside infinitude)
Spontaneously The Giver flashed out the thought
Of the world: more love for the Loved One, more joy to share.
The Spirit fleshed out the thought and the world evolved.
The Loved One seized creation; his anguished soul
Burned to give, to return an excess of love.
Intoxicated he embraced the unfolding Gift,
Virgin wooed and loved and won, a Bride
And joyful Daughter, a Garden Locked, a Well
Of Living Water. "At last, my flesh and bone!
Companion fit! Cost though a world of pain,
The cost were slight to magnify his Name."
    Thus in the living edge Godsong flows
    Ancient and young, youngest where the Spirit blows ...

Were Truth as young as the edge of time, Truth
Would strike like a meteor, transfigure face
And heart. The rushing Wind, the Flames, the Sound,
Would fuel mightily the "fire cast
On the earth." Fire rampant to feed its flame,
Exhaust itself in one vast conflagration,
Depleted of the least spark, entombed as charred
Flesh: "Loved his own to the end." The Bride
Once poor as Cinders, flames an eternal jewel.
In Lover's imitation the Bride floods
The poorest with the riches of her heart. Poor,
Abandoned, an ecstasy of joy, She awaits
    Rich in trust. Godsong eternal flows,
    Spirals in love and beauty where the Spirit blows ...

Bridgeland

Whatever else: bridges are for crossing.
Enjoy/ignore their handsome lines they connect
Two points and the hidden shore's my aim. The BridgeMan
Is sound; proof are the myriad voices that call
Me there, call with incessant joy, singing
Of what they see, who fills their minds, who makes
Them ever new as he is new, the GodMan
Building his newborn family of Bridgeland folk.
Cross over, my easily captured soul, gazing
To admire the faces near or the hills remote,
Itching to linger, to sketch or scribble. BridgeMan
Has called me out of darkness, no more to walk
Blindly idling lost on Bridgeland, nor trembling
In a haunted house. Cross over! No pipe-dreams indulge,
Scrap mundane schemes! Be impatient as GodMan
For my salvation. The Bridge race will not believe
The Bridgeland connects with Paradise. Trusting
In him means moving on, losing our pitch
On the Bridge, its reassurance, our nest. O BridgeMan,
Compel our hearts! Bridgeland will sink: lost
Its purpose, lost all hope of the homeward crossing …

Mam's Philosophy

"It's brilliant! I'm getting
Younger and younger, lighter
And lighter, higher and higher!
It must be true, Dom Bruno affirms it so!
Benedicamus Domino!"

I know you feel younger and lighter,
    Eyes getting brighter.
But ageing's a fact not feeling:
    Fortune is wheeling.

"It's playful delectation
    Not silly deception."

Loving's God's intimate beauty;
    We tend there by duty.
Christ in his heavenly splendour
    Invites to the Father.

"The Phoenix Fire renews me
    All blithe and frisky!"

There in his beauty and brightness
    Drink joy of his goodness.
There there is youth worth awaiting,
    God's love unabating.

Rainbow Leaves

That you could see the rainbow leaves
    On the peach
    And the nectarine!

Seen through the windowpane, framed
    In the white
    Like Fairy Queen.

Tints curved and pointed sway
    On the breeze,
    A sunset scene.

Store up such dreams; blue fingered days
    Encroach
    And a harsh routine.

My crudely fashioned jewels accept
    As warmth
    For the winters lean.

Schooled by loveliness joy lives
    In the soul
    And the heart's ravine.

The Scarecrow

Blackbirds nestle within my breast, sing
And chatter and seek no loftier beatitude.
O wicked scarecrow! Useless! I should be King
Of this small field, master of solitude.
One simple task is mine: scare this field
Of vermin. This done the crop will swiftly grow.
My Master should be severe; a weighty yield
He should demand with vengeance. And rightly so.
O stuffed and coward heart! The song is sweet
Of birds. You idly listen till daylight fades.
I should be free, alone, to watch discrete,
A terror to every foe whose charm persuades,
    Whose song can kill. Naked stands my plight:
    O Flame-Eyed, I feel you gaze stern in the night ...

The Kingfisher

I was walking downcast through the woods
Upon the mouldering earth arched
Over by the black entanglement
Of trees when a Kingfisher rose
From the waters and I watched it
Sparkling through the black crossword
Puzzle. Then suddenly the Sun burst
Through the entangled boughs upon me
And I fell Sunstruck. A violent
Ray ran down the abyss of my mind
Leaving my braincells bleeding like honeycomb.
The Sunray kindled my abyss and burnt
The black arches of night. I knelt up
And saw mankind's whole life issuing into
One bloodred Sunset of happiness.

Old Anna

She prays alone (the dimlit
Church is empty)
Rapt in the holy sacrifice immense.
O what fantastic love
Laid on for one old woman!
    And the world is asleep.

A million suns of grandeur
Guide her heartbeat
Hiding behind her face so old and grey,
Its form and smoothness lost,
Concealed from worldly wisdom.
    And the world is asleep.

True loveliness lies hidden:
Grace and goodness
Hide within our Eucharistic feast.
She opens up her heart:
There God pours love and beauty.
    And the world is asleep ...

The Shulammite

I am black
Like the tents of Kedar.
I am black
Like the shades
On the hills at night.
I am scorched by the sun,
Dark like the curtains
Of Solomon's throne.
I am a rose of Sharon,
A lily of the valley.
His voice is my mirror
And his voice is true.
And he comes to me
Leaping across the mountains
Like a gazelle or a young stag.
And he calls to me,
"Arise my fair one and come away!"
And his call is in the heart;
And his face
Is beautiful in my heart …

Susan

My name is Susan.
I live in the slums.
I eat baked beans every day.
I hear the trains go by.
I am cold in the winter.
I hold my hands out to this people.
My name is Abel
Whom you slew in the country.
My name is Jesus
Whom you crucified in the City.
My blood drips in the dirty teacups,
In the fallen plaster,
In the slum-foul air.
My blood drips in the unseen heart.
I am your little sister
Whom you cannot see.
I am near you:
Put your arm around me!

Snowflakes

"O world of snowflakes, falling, wheeling!
Exquisite patterns drifting, fusing!
Our hearts are futile, snowflakes swirled
Within a cold and pointless world;
And all our days the fires remain
To mock our hopes, drive men insane ..."

Poetry betrays with a wink
Befriending who spurn man's saving link!
Does inspiration grope for aid,
Or pluck a flower to quickly fade?
Does it not seize on truth itself,
And hold it fast with love itself?
Is it not worthy to guide the hand
That marks the way to a higher land?
But atheistic poets grab
And guess and a wounded world they stab.
Their inspiration's a broken horn;
Their snowflakes melt at the break of morn.

O pray for Rilke who left God's narrow way
To roam broad moors, a dismal emigré.

The Knight's Song

    "Lady Rainbow, my Rose!"
Cried the Knight. "Divinely blue,
Immortal white, more joyful than yellow
Flowers adance on the greenest meadow;
Rose in a rusty helmet, true
If the wandering knight be untrue; gay
As sunlit highlands; joy in a deluged soul
Drowned in a flood of self-reproach, prey
To a score of greeds, anxious hole
Of glory tangible of despair;
Lost at sea while sin devours,
Sinking I gaze on the clouds of shifting lies
Stunned at the mystic Arc, her beauty flowers
Shimmering through our feckless skies:
Hope! Hope for my dwindling days,
Hope when the mind's a thorny meadow,
Hope in the heart of failure, Rainbow
Spangling my disenchanted days,
    O Lady Rainbow, my Rose!"

The Olive Tree

Twilight. Time to sleep, to dream,
Forget the busy world. How gleam
Those stars free and far away
From earthly tumult, dust and sway.

Listen! Steps I hear again.
Silence sharpens round these men,
These four, here they often come
To pray beyond the city's hum.

Darkness. Gravely one leaves his friends.
With power a heavy hand descends;
He falls, crushed, oppressed by hate;
He claws the dirt: how deadly his fate!

Starlight (tangled in my aged
And twisted boughs like silver laid
With skill) outlines his haggard face
And sparkles where blood has left its trace.

Silent Birds

Four of the clock and no birds sing. Still dark
The starlit treetops. The chestnut coterie
Of silent birds awaits the magic spark
Of morn to rise and glitter across the lea.
Then so must I: "Rise not before the dawn!"

So Wisdom spoke of old; and old is young
With him whose truth continues true. Advice
Reluctantly embraced, impatient among
The boughs and wind my cold and ingrained vice.
Yet hear I must: "Rise not before the dawn!"

O birds more wise than I. By instinct's decree
You sleep or sing; you brightly toil or bear
The pains that pearl the silent heart. O flee,
My soul to freedom! Like birds abandon care.
Let Wisdom rule: "Rise not before the dawn!"

Tread patiently. Love's hour matures by law
The counterpart eternal of seed that guides
The total mystery home. In him no flaw
Can mar this enterprise while the heart abides
In watchful prayer: "Rise not before the dawn!"

Origin of Flame

Galaxies emergent in the Idea,
Orbit of genesis of stars:
Flashpoint in perfect number
Rendered symbiosis eternal
Free of division from flame's
Origin to flower
Where the still and the furious intersect ...

Distinct systems involve
Stars within stars; intercies
Of vast brown devoid of vision,
Flashpoint, future,
Whose vital feelings flame
Static in still memory
Mirror of unchanging tomorrow ...

And we have seen its flashpoint
As of Elected Children
Full of gravity,
Traversing space inaccessible
On destined elipse, (wheel
Lightyears over Blindspot): Flamelilies
Brilliant shimmering in the Idea ...

God's Dependence

On whom the worlds depend dependency's
Unthinkable of him, yet freely he knocked.
At the dawn of mankind's freedom he humbly stood,
He waited for a human welcome that must be free:
Where there is choice consent is needed; respect
For the creature's heart obliged Omnipotence,
While love beyond conceiving risked all and stood.
The Lover is overawed by the one he loves;
Perfection has paralysed him. "Unruly love's"
No part in God but here "one tress of hair"
Has flamed such magnitudes of love that God
Is vanquished, knocks at the bridal chamber and waits:
"Yes, as you have said so be it." The girl
Calmed her turbulent mind in the Spirit's power.
That "Yes" unlocked God's heart. Without consent
Dawn could not have challenged the reign of night;
Spring could not have conquered mountains of snow.
Seeds a million deep in the frozen earth
Would still be seeds unselfrevealed, unknown
In God. One "Yes" till the end of time. "Yes"
In a trillion heart to a love-dependant God.

The Rusty Plough

The plough on the headland rests in the brambles now.
Unused its handsom share is eaten with rust.
"Why do you lean here idly with hours of light,
With horses standing by and a field to plough?"

"No man has called me." The world has an anguished brow
For the part that suffers and the part that dies in Lust.
The many facets of man have need of light
But the power of the soil needs taming: there's a field to plough.

It's in the furrow the rust-flakes yield; the plough
And the blade begins to shine. The constant thrust
To the future, the fight with fear and slought, delight
In a certain Face gives relish for a field to plough.

The plough must be invested while Spring is now.
Plunge in the soil, cut through the tangled crust!
The sower needs you, the harvest needs your might.
Let not the people languish: there's a field to plough.

A Face still haunts the rusting share of the plough,
A Love outwaiting the heart's dark wanderlust.
Yoke up to grace, harness the dwindling light,
Cleave the furrow: there's a field to plough.
Envoi:
    Now every soul's a ploughshare
        And every life's a field;
    And every field is broadcast
        That splendid might be the yield.

Serenade To Night

Poetry is stillnesses of the flame
Snuffed out by harsh day. Night's the flint
Of rekindling. The flame lives in darkness.
Profundities are her face, the stars her voice.
In the day I do not remember her, I forget
Her livingness. In day's brutality
I weep for the bright eyed Night. In daylight my soul
Spreads like oil over worthless things, seeps
Into crevices, soaks into dross, one
With the tinder of a twinkling conflagration
When the last trumpet sounds. Vile attachment!
Oh this whore heart, unfaithful, cruel!
And the Night is never far. Faithful, serene,
She sooths my anxieties, my stupidity
She schools again and again. The sheer beauty
Of Night, the flame of the Spirit of love living
In the hollowness of my empty well, this heart,
This hole-in-the-air. "And Night shall be your light."
And the poems that drop cheap as pebbledash
Are groaning exiles from the holy face of God ...

Hunger For Recognition

We hunger for recognition: by ugliest means
And fair lifelong this hunger drives us, builds
Cities of greed or pomp, tinsel or power;
Dichotomy of soul, force unknown
Hidden in the Trojan Horse, a Jekyll and Hyde
Who never meet, who frustrate the healing of grace.
Sobered by this split we humble our hearts
Fearful that unbeknown our Trojan Horse
May drop agents of the prince of darkness. My friend
Of joyful mien has died lamented by all.
We reeled to find his Hydeself, his chosen books
Which filled his room. We never met this Hyde
Indulging pornography, cesspools drank
Where God in his Temple dwells. Lay not this sin
Against him! Hunger for recognition drove
His lower self to this; drove his social
Self to joyful and winning ways. The two
Were miles apart, an adolesent he lived
And died in morbid fascination for lust.
Jesus, may he rest in peace, 'know
As we are known' and in the Father's love
His soul's true hunger find satisfaction as son.

I Am Two Barley Loaves ...

Not worth the mention among this multitude.
Food for a boy my ambitions have no more force.
Why not feed them with food from nothing? With him
The effort's equal; say but the word and manna
Will cover the ground like snow, quail will fall
From the sky. Yet who would question him? His way
Is awesome. Someone wiser than Solomon
Is here. His works reveal his wisdom in ages
Still to come. He chooses the weak and little,
Things of no account; discrete his ways
Not showy. I remain my humble self yet feed
Five thousand famished souls hungering for God.
I remain a single meal for a lad hidden
From thousands who ate their fill of me. Happy
To be his creature single or multiplied,
Known or unknown, despised or crowned with gold.
I know myself and am known by him. "A body
You gave me. Behold I come to do your will!"
I am two barley loaves; I am; I am not;
I am a rose or silence; I am an anguished
Heart, a lamb on the fire; I am indifference ...

Jew's Harp

I'm no great shakes, only a Jew' harp,
A give-away, however great my Muse. Not
That I would blame him, the twangy sound
Is me. How (and if) he plucks my humble harp's
Beyond discernment. It's more a hope. I desire
No other and no less inspiration. To speak
Of him whom I desire builds up desire. I
Shape my mind, unravel the tangled track.
Perhaps desire is prayer, hope abandonment
To his power. Music is not his need but an open
Heart: "I will speak to her heart." Why
Would you speak? My amazement grows in leaps
And bounds that Starmaker's eager to speak
To us, is overwhelmingly concerned about me!
I see magnitudes. He sees each speck and disregards
The mighty cosmos: he sees me and loves me! Is that
Too much to believe? Does the world in me
Laugh? A Jew's harp is comical, no one performs
Without derision. The galaxies are a speck
To tip the scales but the heart's his rapturous
Kingdom; "We will make our dwelling in you. Your
Heart's the Spirit's Temple of Fire. Fire is my
Substance. I am all speech, all silence, timeless
Resonance of love. Slain but alive I am one
Ambition: passionate to sing on the tiniest harp!"

Hitler and the Treasures in Dark Places

Can you see now the "treasures" God
Prepared for himself in the "dark places" provided
By your evil genius, the "hoards in secret"?
How do you feel? Hoodwinked you played the game
Of Satan to full extent. You had your reward,
You tasted power as no man before. You toppled
In ignominious flames. You live on our lips
A shadowy immortality of little
Value to you. But the jewels were never brighter
Than those you made. Unprecedented the hate
In debasing the image of God, in savagery
So uncontrolled, so efficient the system of killing,
The martyrs were never martyred with such polished skill
Like that! So when the black horror has gone
And the jewels sparkle with everlasting joy
We glimpse something of the mystery of God, his vision,
His terrifying decision to give you life,
To let you prance on the world's stage, to crush
The grapes of Eshcol, the beautiful children of God ...

The Great Unknown

(Sounds like my own biography, the great
Unknown, unread with avidity!
Who cares for vulgar success, a flash in the sky,
When noble oblivion smiles on my earthly course?)
Warfare thrives in secret; unknown my part,
A fiend in the shadows, gay in a shady treetop
God's sniper selects his victims: King Innocens,
Generalissimo Turkey of the elegant strut,
Miss World of ninety seven summers flushed
With modest victory still. Confident
My aim and true. As corpse on corpse falls
Compassion glows within me; the soul released
Soars to judgement and there God's sniper sheds
His weapons and, Christlike, weeps for a fallen race ...

The Welsh Jeweller

The Jeweller fashions in her
Intense circle of light
A brooch for a neckband, a ring
For a bride. Each word, each dash,
Each image chiselled with care,
Sculptured to polished art.

A new world sparkles, lives
In the womb-like circle of light
Where heart and fist, face
And the feeling of life emerge
As love of sculptured thought
Shapes beauty, jewels of the heart.

God too is a maker of jewels,
The poor (princely paid
A rip-off in flesh) who live
Circled in love, cast care
To the brooding Spirit, rejoice
In beauty: grace-sculptured heart.

For Vuyelwa Carlin

Set Apart for Splendour

Something close to nothing;
Worse: dust in sin;
This body of death, this wretchedness,
Set apart for splendour;
Designated to offer fire,
A pleasing odour
Like galbanum, onycha and stacte,
And like the fragrance
Of frankincense in the tabernacle.
Consecrated to handle the Holy Things,
To offer trembling the cup of destiny.
Set apart as holy
To serve with hallowed fire
The watchful heart one flowing doxology.
Dust transfigured
In ever increasing brightness
Till like bronze mirrors our faces
Reflect his Glory whose eyes
Are flames of fire
Among the splendours of the saints ...

To Be Here

To be here
Where the Light streams;
To be here
Covered by the shining Cloud;
To be here always
Where the majestic voice speaks;
To be here
On the mountain gazing up at you,
Jesus, the Light more beautiful
Than the billion-star creation streaming
Through your face!

Easter Island

Who dwells here?
An Ego in solitude,
Worming down
To its nothingness?
Ever more intrigued
By self's totem pole,
Admired from every angle,
Circumdanced in worship?
That which is-not
Excludes
He-who-is,
The mystery which elevates,
Spirals the soul above the Island's
Solitude, above the silence,
Above where Christ enthroned
Is Mystery
Worshipped, worthy of unending
Adoration,
Of Paschal Joy
In selfforgetfullness.
Who dwells here?

Deadly Nightshade

Pluck up this deadly nightshade symbol of an age,
Worshipped, fought for, drug of a thirsting world.
Oh for the depths of God! For the Spring
Flowing with life eternal! To cleanse the beasts
Of darkness who kill for twopence, who love for lust
And violence. Dehumanised by lovelessness,
Cast on the streets like offal their unfledged soul
Finds dignity in the passions of the brute, in power
Over weaklings, defiance of a corrupt and heartless world.
We drug them with poisoned waters. What fatuous rights
We invent, titles to pollute the pure! Our necks
Will bow to millstones cast in a sea of fire.
Oh for the long-forsaken fountain to gush
In the night, for Wisdom to raise her voice in the streets!
Jesus, greater than wisdom, living and true,
Light streaming from your face, hear
This cry of dereliction! We hunger to save
And cherish and the world goes gun in hand. Oh Eyes
Of flame within, flash on the tortured world!
Man, priest of creation, cheap as dirt,
Gunned down bleeds in the gutter! "In him we live
And move and have our being." Held in his hands
We love or hate, kill or care. War
Of ages; our deatiny we forge in symbols:
Deadly Nightshade, the Lily and the Rose.

The Carnival

The world is a Carnival, the heart of the world.
All its life is here, its longings, its memories.
Here is the merrygoround, the music, the lights,
The laughter. Here are people out for excitement.
All that is young and gay, the dance and the thrills.
But God was not in the Carnival, he was not
In the earthquake nor in the thunder and dread. God
Was in silence. My heart was wrapped in layers
Of flesh. All of the senses cried for life,
An act in time, a pinprick of pleasure; strung
Together one felt alive in satisfaction
Till boredom intervened. And the Carnival
Turned sour and loud, a burden crushing the soul.
Why did you call me out of the Carnival
Into your marvellous light? The mercies of God
I will not cease to sing. The mystery of God
I will not cease to exalt. The blinding force
Behind the exploding cosmos, the almighty surge
Flinging out forever's a tiny image
Of God. So I watch the stars with joy. Night
Hands on to night its silent Carnival
Of light, the merryground, the unending thrill.
Here before the awesome explosion of life
My heart sings in the Carnival of Love …

Mystery

For all my abuse and anger
The world will march on not one whit better!
My Pharisee still rants
Blinded by windy indignation.
Always till the final doom
(One bomb too big or a frozen planet)
The world is a school of virtue,
A temple of the hidden God where love
Grows in the scourge of chaos.
The Spirit broods on darkness; his passion,
Maternal fruitfulness,
Teems with newness, new life springs
In the Spirit's unfelt warmth.
O be my sun, my carefree summer
Days! Be my day
And night, my winter however long!
The end, the end is all!
And the end is mystery, the plan hidden,
Sparkling before the world,
The unfolding scheme of our salvation
Woven from the skein of time.
New life in multitudes, new life
For the passionate, humble heart.
The Father's fathomless power outpouring
Yearns for a contrite heart:
"Fill me with joy and gladness, this body
Shall thrill with pride!" O come,
God creative, burning for lands
To conquer, to lavish treasures
Of love, divine, inexhaustible self,
In the trusting, aching heart!

The Field of Silence

My investments are too divided, weakened.
My gold is too spread out, little
Heaps in silly interests and little
Satisfaction. I will relinquish
Shares in trivial commodities,
Amass my whole talent of gold
For one total project: treasure
Hidden in a Field. O Field
Of Silence unexcavated! Seen
And soon forgotten, treasures immense.
Sung of by trusty men who delved
A lifetime in peace, enriched their mind
With faith, their lips with burning praise.
The presence of God so vivid this Field
Gives unstinting, a sunrise so fair
All other sunups sink in shame,
Dead planets stripped of glamour. Go,
All little things! The Field is free,
No limits to my greed! Day
And night, healthy or ill, intense
At work or leisured, God's will wrapped
In silence is found in the treasure Field.
God of the silent heart turns Flame ...

Snake-City

Down the centre of the sunny cloister
Waddling like a tired, triumphant washer-
Woman the mallard goes heading her string
Of fluffy offspring chirping gaily, skitty,
Flitting inquisitively, a nervous ganglion
Of innocence. Each year the mallard nests
(Appropriately!) between the mounds where the bones
Of the old monks rest. When her ducklings play
In the lily pond (a sheer delight to watch)
She stands erect head pointed upwards on guard
Watching the peaceful blue whence death strikes:
Kestrel, jay and magpie, an evil trio,
Wait impatiently a meal of duckling!
A swift dive, silence, alarm, and her brood
Is minus one. She saves, say, two a year;
Nature's law not love. Somewhere a snake
Eating its tail symbolises nature
Well. Devouring itself perpetuates
Itself. If humans live for the baser pleasures
We revert to the cyclic snake: we kill to augument
Our wealth, our power, our ego. Life's a duck's life.
Kestrel, Jay and Magpie Esq attack
Youth with claws exploiting their weakness, run
Abortion mills, grow fat on suicide clinics.
Connivance across the board spreads the cancer.
Politicians pander, health insurance
Bribes, coaches on tour debase gratis
En route lusting for infants, judges, wink,
Mrs Jay leads pastors by the nose;
Apathetic in wealth the rest of us view
Trousered apes in Fleet Street strip cartoons.
Love can break the vicious circle. God
Is Love but him we have mocked and cast outside
The walls. "As a hen gathers her brood and yet
You would not! O Snake-City ...."

An Ear For Silence

Souls have inward senses: we see yet mean
We know; we hear yet understand; we feel
Yet mean we think; we "taste that the Lord is sweet"
Yet mean the experience of the spirit, the heart's
Persuasion that God's indwelling is real and good,
We relish his living presence, the Love that ran
To meet us broken on the road of life. "My one
Desire: to dwell in the house of God forever."
God is our home. We abide in him. He lives
In us. No space between us though we are a mite
(The all of the poorest widow) and he riches
Inexhaustible; we are small
And he inhabits space and beyond, time
And beyond; we feel our wretchedness and lower
Our eyes in shame, his pardon gives life like spring,
His burning sanctity no longer slays,
Maternal-like his bosom, paternal his arms.
O sea of God, give me an ear for silence!
Silence, the aura of Being, stillness and pulse
Of Love, flowing, ebbing, igniting. Cleansed
In the cataclysmic torrents of Jesus' Blood
Our hearing opens, is seized by Triune music,
Entranced by silence while timeless eons unfold ...

Not To Other gods My Glory

Jesus, put fire in my worship!
That it may please God, say my utmost,
Bring to acknowledge him my total being.
He draws me in secret, I feel it.
I must take stock, the thing is urgent.
All my intelligence, my will, my feelings
Force me to conversion,
To change my course; time's no longer
A luxury spread out for the rich, lavish
Before me. Behind, my footprints
Concentrate annihilating
Time, contracting space, colliding memories.
My past's the edge of tomorrow.
My final stretch swings into vision.
Homeward bound: the thrill of the Unknown unending ...

One God, One Substance only;
And we but accidental, not needful
To him. Since Love is Substance, joy is Being's
Act, its only Act. Creation's needless
But Love has spoken. Love has burst its boundaries,
Outpouring itself in Glory:
"Not to other gods my Glory.
Not for your greatness I made you: in Love I chose you;
Not merit but Love's my meaning."
Our Substance cannot change, his meaning
Stands eternal. Jesus, put Fire in routine!
My worship must be fitting,
Fire for the God of Fire! Homeward
Bound: to plunge in the Substance of Fire unending ...

Pilgrim of the Interior

"The Kingdom is within you. Follow me."
My journey's well trodden ground. Where all have walked
To find him so must I go. The road is thick
With travellers, a solemn joy prevails. Yet all
Are blind: "We walk by faith not sight." We trust
The One who called to silence, who went before,
Through death and resurrection, to an unknown Land.
Our homeland is in the heavens and in the heart.
The Land is nowhere. We seek no land or place.
The Kingdom is a reign of peace; all hearts at peace
And every yearning resolved. He is our peace
Beyond the anguish of time and martial law.
He is our freedom: insidious darkness, sin,
The sting of death, plucked from the heart. A new
Creation of stars, a higher cosmos of hearts
Spin out brilliant from him. He is our hope
And our salvation. Silent we follow lost
In mystery. Our pilgrimage unfolds more
By trust than steps, desire than deeds, love
Than ancient maps. The call's unique; the Cross
Calls to the depths of God: "There will I speak
To your heart and you shall know that I am God."
"Deep echoes deep" in the pilgrim's candid heart.
The pilgrimage descends till Christ presents
His pilgrims "clothed in parted tongues of Fire":
The Father's love's in all and all are One.

Locked Out

Wretchedness and grace are lock and key.
Our humbling poverty invites All-Power
Whose presence completes his work in a wealth of peace.
The wars of difference find resolution here:
The Oneness at the core of Wisdom. Our nought, our guilt,
Our death were fearsome indeed, evils beyond
All comprehension were God not Life and Love.
The mystery of the lock, the Locked Garden, the Black
Shulammite are solved in the avalanche
Of grace. Through grace the lock is opened, a world
Of breathless vision swings into view: Eden
Lost now found sublimer still at one
With the soul, its ground, its atmosphere, its sun.
God is the blazing core and I the Bush
        On Fire. Where Christ's dire poverty had shocked
        Torrents unpriced gush in the Garden Locked ...

The Prayer of Hope

Blindness may be our greater good: "See
That nothing worse befall you." Blinded from birth
Was no sin. Seeing, enticements are vivid,
Multiply. Better cast dust in his eyes
Than leave him seeing to walk blindly to sin.
Better to sow uncertainty, doubts
Of being special, exception to the rule,
Than approve (with priestly state) and watch him pass
To death and judgement. Better judgement face
With tax collector's prayer, with diffidence,
Than with the Pharisee calmly assume
Acceptance. Compassion's bread stales when love
Is blind. You let him walk (gave him your staff)
A perilous track in peace of mind to a cliff ...

Was it Christ-like to say "Go in peace,"
and omit, "Sin no more"? Not even, "Try."
The power of Christ, the power of virtue, slew
Death and sin, "the sting of death." To believe
And reject this power is failure to respond.
The medicine of life cannot fail: death
Is vanquished. "The death he died he died to sin.
In him's no shadow of sin. In him we live.
The life I live I live in the Son of God
Who loved me and died for me. Seated above
With Christ I bear in my flesh the wounds of love."

The Kingdom of God

O the superior joy of faith,
Fire, of "God a consuming Fire!"
Thomas, how could you doubt! How could
They extol your snub reducing to lies
The witness of honest folk! They saw
Christ risen, the tomb smashed!
They saw the seed dead, saw
Deep, divine life spring
Immortal, an explosion of love, joy
Singing on the roads of the world! Your sulk
Aborted the child of grace. Christ
Upbraided your unbelieving heart.
Cast out fear! Let the child be born
To soar: "of such is the Kingdom of God!"

Concert of Fire

I am a song on the lips of God.
A song has slight existence,
A second? but yet flows on;
    And its cause is special: love and joy.

I become, I sound, I linger on the lips
Of God because he loves me.
Creates he nothing save love
    Conceived: Love's the fountain of life.

A Singer in love breaks forth in song
And his song, his voice, his creation,
Magnify his bliss.
    The loved one lives on the lips of Love.

Forever my Love, my God, will sing.
My being is thought singing
One with the fabric of Love.
    I'm a note ever new, a song to his Love.

O for the will of God most pure!
One in his mind and willing,
Blending my voice in his heart:
    Concert of Fire, One Singer, One Song!

Flashpoint

Time is a flashpoint; and in a flash it will
Not be. In the flash is the matter of a moment
Too weak to endure. Hovering somewhere between
A past of timeless shadows, a future as infinite
And uncontrolled our flashpoint home glimmers,
St Elmo's Fire, Will-o-the-wisp, all
Our wonder and woe. Here we are concentrated,
Curled up in Little Ease, a green sheathed
Rosebud where choices have deceptive faces.
God grounds successive flashpoints maintaining core
Identity all unfolding in him, foundation
Of order, goal of every atom and soul.
God's too-much beauty kills: this whole foundation
Breaks in, breaks the senses too paltry flashpoint
And kills choice. The soul is saturated,
Divine foundation claiming the whole ground,
The whole landscape transfigured light. Flashpoints
Frizzle out, Will-o-the-wisp's paltry
Pleasures scatter in shame. Too-much Beauty
Absorbs one's whole freedom, choices are as dead
As flashpoint carrion. Life's moment is too narrow.
O the mystery of life, exhaustive flash without point.
Life is the flower of dying, unsought for peace,
"Its flashes are flashes of fire, a vehement flame!"

Truth and Trust

Ignorance is a subtle defence where trust is dead.
Privacy unassailable; starvation, death,
Preferred to capitulation to truth. Besiegers
Vanquished by evasion. Truth unwelcomed
Cannot force an entry, must humbly knock,
And does. "The truth would set you free." Free
Of what? Freedom from uneasy deeds
Darkly perceived unworthy of the light;
"And Adam and Eve hid from the face of God."
We hide in a glass prison our shameful self
(Forgetful how transparent the whole game is)
Pretend, avoid the light, walk on alone ...

The sceptic is proud of his lack (unrecognised)
Of trust. Trust is a bridge to another's heart.
Trust reaches out to smiles, to goodness; creates
Life by trusting; is not repulsed when the face
Is granit. Trust is irrepressible love,
God's image in us, building bridges, linking
Heart to heart, the world one fabic woven
Of living strands, time's human tapestry,
Alive from Adam to the final trumpet's call.
O God of the living, break our prison of doubt
And isolation, our prison of shame! Call
The famished heir, call splendour from the sty!